Words to the Wise

Books by Thomas Szasz

Pain and Pleasure
The Myth of Mental Illness
Law, Liberty, and Psychiatry
Psychiatric Justice
The Ethics of Psychoanalysis
The Manufacture of Madness
Ideology and Insanity
The Age of Madness (ed.)
The Second Sin
Ceremonial Chemistry
Heresies
Karl Kraus and the Soul Doctors
Schizophrenia
Psychiatric Slavery
The Theology of Medicine
The Myth of Psychotherapy
Sex by Prescription
The Therapeutic State
Insanity
The Untamed Tongue
Our Right to Drugs
A Lexicon of Lunacy
Cruel Compassion
The Meaning of Mind
Fatal Freedom
Pharmacracy
Liberation by Oppression
Words to the Wise

Words to the Wise

A Medical-Philosophical Dictionary

Thomas Szasz

Transaction Publishers
New Brunswick (U.S.A.) and London (U.K.)

This book is printed on acid-free paper that meets the American National Standard for Permanence of Paper for Printed Library Materials.

Library of Congress Catalog Number: 2003053136
ISBN: 0-7658-0217-1
Printed in the United States of America

Library of Congress Cataloging-in-Publication Data

Szasz, Thomas Stephen, 1920-
Words to the wise : a medical-philosophical dictionary / Thomas Szasz.
p. cm.
Includes bibliographical references and indexes.
ISBN 0-7658-0217-1 (cloth : alk. paper)
1. Psychiatry—Philosophy—Dictionaries. 2. Mental illness—Philosophy—Dictionaries. I. Title.

RC437.5.S934 2004
616.89'001—dc21 2003053136

Contents

Preface and Acknowledgments

The human mind abhors the absence of explanation. Most people, most of the time, have (what they consider) an understanding of everything that concerns them. Of course, the understanding of the child or uneducated person is likely to be wrong. The educated, respectable adult's understanding is likely to be incomplete and, more often, erroneous. To make matters worse, it is likely to be supported as truth and wisdom by religious and scientific authority, intellectual fashion, and social convention.

Despite enormous social pressure for a shared perspective on how the world works and how we ought to live, it is no exaggeration to say that every person's understanding, not only of himself, but of the world about him, is different from every other person's. At the same time, harmonious social relations require a large measure of commonality—the same language and religion, an agreed upon system of measures, shared views about family relations, work, disease, and death. This is why the group—especially if it is or believes itself to be under attack—values erroneous consensus more highly than contested truth. The quest for truth tends to be divisive. "An ounce of loyalty," Arthur Koestler aptly remarked, "is worth a pound of brains."

Everyone knows that ignorance and false understanding abound, yet the typical person is confident that what he "knows" is so. Such a mistakenly self-confident person will be unable to overcome his ignorance. We can propose an answer to someone who asks a question. But if he believes he already knows the answer, he can only preach or teach. Zealots—religious, political, medical—"know." They ask no questions, ponder no problems, entertain no uncertainties.

The problem I address in this book is intrinsic to the human condition. The American humorist, Josh Billings (Henry Wheeler Shaw, 1818-1885), described it this way: "The trouble with people is not what they don't know but that they know so much that ain't so." This problem is in perennial need of being remedied. From Montaigne and La Rochefoucauld, to Kraus, Bierce and Mencken, philosophers and writers have done so, with brevity and levity, deflating error as if it were hot air filling an empty balloon, needing only to escape when provided a ready exit.

Throughout my life, I have tried to avoid Billings's warning about "knowing what ain't so." Many of my books are devoted to exposing what ain't so about mental illness and psychiatry. In this book I apply the same skeptical spirit to a broad range of subjects, from birth to death.

I am keenly aware of the wisdom of Jonathan Swift's admonition, "It is useless to attempt to reason a man out of a thing he was never reasoned into." Still, I persist in the belief that a man, seeing another reason himself out of error, may decide to do the same for himself.

I thank my family, friends, and fans who, in various ways, contributed to this book. I am especially indebted to my brother George, my daughter Margot, son-in-law Steve, and Peter Uva, senior librarian at Upstate Medical University, for their generous and steadfast help. Alice Michtom, Keith Hoeller, Nicolas Martin, Jeffrey Schaler, Mira de Vries, and Roger Yanow read all or parts of the manuscript and offered much constructive criticism. David Ramsay Steele has kindly permitted me to reuse some material from my book, *The Untamed Tongue* (La Salle, Illinois: Open Court, 1990). Finally, I thank Michael Paley, my editor at Transaction Publishers, for his conscientious, knowledgeable, and sympathetic work on the manuscript.

A

Addiction

Giving oneself an addictive drug is a crime; receiving it from a government agent called an "addiction specialist" is a treatment.

* * *

If a person ingests a drug prohibited by legislators and claims that it makes him feel better, that proves that he is an addict.

If he ingests a drug prescribed by psychiatrists and claims that it makes him feel better, that proves that mental illness is a biomedical disease.

* * *

When Judaism in Spain was prohibited and Catholicism prescribed, many Jews became Catholics. This was called "religious conversion."

Today, when heroin in the United States is prohibited and methadone is prescribed, heroin addicts are often turned into methadone addicts. We call this "medical treatment."

* * *

Actors and athletes, with superlative control over their bodies, are paraded as victims of an insidious illness—drug addiction—that robs them of their ability to control their craving for drugs. Most Americans prefer that illusion to the reality that such persons are guilty of the four deadly sins: lust, pride, gluttony, and greed.

* * *

"I regard relationship addiction as a definable, diagnosable and treatable *disease process,*" declares Robin Norwood, author of the 1985 best seller, *Women Who Love Too Much.*[1]

The popular belief, validated by physicians and politicians, that drug addiction, alcohol addiction, gambling addiction, food addiction, shopping addiction, tobacco addiction, and sex addiction are diseases signifies that we are in the grips of a medical fundamentalism no less bizarre or extreme than the familiar religious fundamentalisms.

Adolescents

Adolescents are not full members of adult society. Hence, it is fallacious to speak of their "dropping out."

Unless a young person exerts himself to become a part of society, he will, without any particular effort, find himself outside of it. That is the bitter lesson J. D. Salinger portrayed so perfectly in *The Catcher in the Rye.*

* * *

Puberty, a biological phenomenon, occurs when the organism has matured enough to procreate. In animals, this coincides with the female's ability to care for its progeny. In humans, too, it coincided at one time, but it no longer does.

The more socially complex and technologically sophisticated society becomes, the wider grows the gap between the age at which its young members develop the biological capacity to procreate and at which they acquire the economic opportunity to act as adults. So long as society fails to take proper account of this fact, it will be plagued by a mounting burden of unwanted and unparented children growing up to be inadequate adults.

Today, teenage parents have the economic, legal, and social burdens of minors, and the responsibilities of adults. Many youngsters may be ready to take charge of their own lives long before they are given the opportunity to do so.

We ought to consider drastically shortening the period of *compulsory education*, allowing people to become full-fledged adults at a younger age, thus facilitating economic independence and its salutary existential side effects.

* * *

We expect adolescents to be capable of using computers and incapable of using drugs, and they often comply.

Advertising

Advertising creates private needs and promises to satisfy them with a product or service.

Demagoguery creates public needs and promises to satisfy them with a social policy or "program."

Agreement

Life would be more harmonious if people were more interested in seeking mutual respect than mutual agreement.

Who needs agreement? The religious zealot, the fanatic nationalist, the doctrinaire professional.

Civilized man is satisfied with respect. His credo is: live and let live.

Alcoholism

Experts assert that the disposition to drink alcohol to excess, leading to "alcoholism," is genetically determined. Once the "alcoholic" knows that, he becomes more, not less, responsible than the non-alcoholic for his drinking and its consequences.

Americans

Americans are the world's most successful manufacturers of trade names, such as Coca Cola, Marlboro, and Prozac. They are also the world's most avid consumers of social and political quackery, from Prohibition and Affirmative Action to the War on Drugs.

* * *

The American mall: a privately owned shopping and entertainment area where the best dressed people are the guards.

Antipsychiatry

Ronald D. Laing (1927-1989), the Scottish "antipsychiatrist," is often believed to have rejected the concept of mental illness and opposed involuntary mental hospitalization and coercive psychiatric treatment. The opposite is the case.

Laing wrote:

1. "Our sanity is not 'true' sanity. Their madness is not 'true' madness.... True sanity entails in one way or another the dissolution of the normal

ego, that false self competently adjusted to our alienated social reality."[2]

2. "*When I certify someone insane, I am not equivocating when I write that he is of unsound mind, may be dangerous to himself and others*, and requires care and attention in a mental hospital."[3]

3. In 1976, Laing's twenty-four-year-old daughter, Fiona, was rejected by her boyfriend. Laing biographer John Clay writes:

> She had "cracked up," and had been found weeping outside a church near the family home. [Committed to a local mental hospital, she is given ECT.] He [Adrian] rang his father up and asked him "in despair and anger" what he was going to do about it. Laing reassured him that he would visit Fiona and "do everything in his power" to ensure that she was not given ECT, but when it came to the crunch, as Adrian Laing relates, all he could say was "Well, Ruskin Place [the family home] or Gartnavel [the "state" mental hospital where Laing received his psychiatric training]—what's the difference?"[4]

* * *

The self-stigmatizing label "antipsychiatry" was the joint product of Ronald D. Laing and David Cooper. In *The Dialectics of Liberation*, Cooper wrote: "The organizing group [of the "Congress on the Dialectics of Liberation," held in London in 1967] consisted of four psychiatrists who...counter-label[ed] their discipline as anti-psychiatry. The four were Dr. R. D. Laing and myself, also Dr. Joseph Berke and Dr. Leon Redler."[5]

Predictably, supporters of coercive psychiatry love to diagnose and dismiss their critics as "antipsychiatrists."

* * *

Lavoisier didn't call himself an "anti-phlogistonian." He simply maintained that phlogiston was the name of an imaginary substance.

Einstein didn't call himself an "anti-etherian." He simply maintained that (the physicist's) ether, like the chemist's phlogiston, was also the name of an imaginary substance.

Luther and Calvin did not call themselves "anti-Christians." They simply rejected the papacy's claims to temporal power and its prevarications about indulgences.

* * *

Michel Foucault (1926-1984), the French psychologist-philosopher-"antipsychiatrist," is also often credited with rejecting the concept of mental illness and opposing the practice of involuntary mental hospitalization. This, too, is inaccurate. Foucault wrote:

> The structural description of mental illness, therefore, would have to analyze the positive and negative signs for each syndrome.... The science of mental pathology cannot but be the science of the sick personality.[6]

> The only thing I can compare this experience to [being intoxicated with LSD] is sex with a stranger... Contact with a strange [male] body affords an experience of the truth similar to what I am experiencing now.[7]

Foucault objected to psychiatric imprisonment *because it was imprisonment* (in an "unjust" capitalist society), *not because it was psychiatric*. In the 1950s, Foucault was a member of the French Communist Party. Literary critic Roger Kimball aptly characterizes Foucault as a man who "never met a revolutionary piety he didn't like. He championed various extreme forms of Marxism, including Maoism...[and] supported the Ayatollah Khomeini."[8]

* * *

It would be nonsensical to call a physician critical of coercions in the name of dermatology an "anti-dermatologist," or a physician critical of coercions in the name of oncology an "anti-oncologist." The fact that it is *not* nonsensical to call a physician critical of coercions in the name of psychiatry an "antipsychiatrist" is evidence that psychiatry is about coercion, not healing.

* * *

In the 1970s, self-styled antipsychiatrists undermined the case against the existence of mental illness and the practice of psychiatric coercions-and-excuses by attributing mental diseases to an "insane society" and claiming success for "treating" such diseases with their particular brand of "therapy."[9]

In the 1990s, self-styled critics of psychiatry undermined the case against the existence of mental illness and the practice of psychiatric coercions-and-excuses by dwelling on the harmfulness of drugging children with Ritalin or adults with Prozac; claiming successful "treatment" for these nonexistent diseases by their particular brand of "empathy and love"; blaming the use of psychiatric drugs on drug companies rather than on psychiatrists, patients, and the relatives of patients; and refusing to recognize that most adults who use psychiatric drugs do so voluntarily, indeed eagerly.[10]

Antipsychotic Drugs

Thomas Szasz (1956):

> [Antipsychotic drugs] function as chemical straitjackets.... When patients had to be restrained by the use of [physical] force—for example, by a straitjacket—it was difficult for those in charge of their care to convince themselves that they were acting altogether on behalf of the patient.... Restraint by chemical means does not make [others] feel guilty; herein lies the danger to the patient.[11]

Artisanship and Artificiality

In the past, most people were engaged in making things others found useful, such as clothing and furniture. They could see and touch the products of their labors and took pride in their work.

Today, while some people are still engaged in providing private services that help others, most people are engaged in providing bureaucratic services that hinder others. In either case, they cannot see or touch the products of their labors. Increasingly, people take pride not in their work but in their hobby, which is likely to be something passive, such as watching baseball on television and being knowledgeable about famous players and the scores of past games.

Thus has modern artificiality replaced premodern artisanship.

Atheism

Webster's defines theism as "belief in the existence of a god or gods; specifically: belief in the existence of one God viewed as the creative source of man and the world who transcends yet is immanent in the world."

Atheism, then, means simply not sharing this belief.

In another sense, theism means religious justification for coercion, persecution, violence, and war, illustrated by the history of killings waged in the name of God; or religious justification for charity, compassion, and love, illustrated by church-based institutions and organizations for relief of human suffering.

Atheism, in this second sense, means rejection of religion as a moral sanction for coercion or a necessary condition for compassion.

In a third sense, atheism is pseudoscientific justification for vilification of and violence against certain individuals and institutions, illustrated by literal violence against them in the Soviet Union and semantic violence against them by militant atheists. For example: Marx calling religion an "opiate," Freud interpreting it as a "neurosis," and Darwin zealot Richard Dawkins attributing it to "memes"—fictitious "self-replicating parasites that infect the mind like computer viruses"—that he invented for the purpose.[12] (See *Memes*)

Atheists

On August 27, 1987, campaigning for the presidency, George Bush held a news conference at O'Hare Airport in Chicago.

> Sherman [Robert I. Sherman, a reporter for the *American Atheist* magazine]: What will you do to win the votes of the Americans who are Atheists?
>
> Bush: I'm pretty weak in the Atheist community. Faith in God is important to me.
>
> Sherman: Surely you recognize the equal citizenship and patriotism of Americans who are Atheists?
>
> Bush: No, I don't know that Atheists should be considered as citizens.... This is one nation under God.[13]

* * *

Many atheists who distrust religion and proclaim their disbelief in God trust psychiatry and proclaim their belief in mental illness. Paul Kurtz—professor of philosophy emeritus at the State University of New York in Buffalo and a leading atheist activist—writes: "The most vitriolic attacks on science in recent decades have questioned its benefits to society.... Many, like Szasz, even deny that there are mental illnesses, though there seems to be considerable evidence that some patients do suffer behavioral disorders and exhibit symptoms that can be alleviated by anti-psychotic drugs."[14]

Autonomy

Autonomy: the paradigmatic heresy, the quintessential affront against authority.

* * *

Autonomy (liberty) is self-directed or, in John Stuart Mill's phrase, "self-regarding": it is exercising one's own powers to act in accordance with one's own free will, for example, resisting a temptation or yielding to it, and assuming responsibility for the consequences.

Right (positive right) is other-directed or "other-regarding": it is lodging a "rightful" claim against others or the state, for example, to payment for services rendered as contractually agreed upon.

Political theorist Anthony de Jasay summarized this important distinction as follows:

> A right confers a benefit on its holder. In order for him to enjoy it, an obligor must fulfill the corollary obligation—which is generally onerous to a degree.... A liberty, on the other hand, is exercised without calling for specific performance by any other party; apart from negative externalities that may be generated by my using it, my liberty is costless to everybody else.... "Costly to others" and "costless to others" are no more alike than black and white.[15]

De Jasay's "liberty to perform" is liberty to exercise one's autonomy.

* * *

There is only one offense against authority: self-control; and only one obeisance to it: submission to control by authority.

The person who controls himself and cares for his own well being has no need of an external authority to protect him from himself. He is his own self-protector.

This renders paternalistic authority unemployed. What is he to do if he cannot control others in the name of protecting them? He could mind his own business. But that is a fatuous answer. Persons satisfied with minding their own business do not aspire to become paternalistic authorities, while persons who become such authorities consider minding other peoples' business their own business and call it "caring" and "assuming responsibility."

Authority needs persons who lack autonomy or whom they can readily deprive of it, such as children, old people, and patients. Hence the ceaseless warfare of authority against autonomy, against suicide, against masturbation, against self-medication, against the proper use of language itself.

* * *

Prior to the Reformation, church and state prohibited the individual from caring for his own soul as he saw fit. Curing souls was the province of the licensed priest. The unlicensed priest and the person who sought his help were considered heretics and were killed.

Today, medicine and state prohibit the individual from caring for his own body. Curing bodies is the province of licensed physicians. Unlicensed healers and their clients are considered drug pushers and drug addicts. The former are incarcerated in prisons, the latter in mental hospitals.

* * *

We are ambivalent about autonomy. We yearn for it when it is taken from us, recoil from it when it is offered to us.

The Forbidden Fruit is the gift of death as much as it is the gift of life.

B

Beauty

Beauty is in the eye of the beholder. Ugliness is in the personality of the beholden.

Behavior

When a dog behaves badly—for example, mauling a baby—we blame it for its behavior and its owner for not having domesticated it.

When a teenager behaves badly—for example, killing and injuring students and teachers in a school shooting—medical experts blame it on everything except him and his parents for not having domesticated him.

* * *

Daniel R. Weinberger, a leading neuroscientist at the National Institute of Health, offered this explanation for a school shooting: "[T]he evidence is unequivocal that the prefrontal cortex of a 15-year-old is biologically immature.... The 15-year-old brain does not have the biological machinery to inhibit impulses in the service of long-range planning."[1]

I commented: "Until recent times, children who reached biological maturity, typically around the age of 13, were treated as adults. Benjamin Franklin was an apprentice printer at age 12, and his brain was evidently well enough developed to plan for the future. Mr. Weinberger's disclaimer—'this brief lesson in brain development is not meant to absolve criminal behavior'—is unpersuasive. Such fashionable neurologizing of bad behavior is destructive of civilized discourse and human relations."[2]

* * *

When and why do we say that a behavior is *caused* rather than *willed*?

We say that chemicals in the brain cause depression and suicide; but we don't say that chemicals in the ovaries or testicles cause lust and marriage.

Chemicals in our bodies incline us toward certain behaviors. Inclinations give us options, to engage in or abstain from certain behaviors. Absent hunger or lust, there is no temptation to eat or copulate. Absent depression (or disability, old age, etc.), there is no temptation to kill oneself.

Self-discipline enables us to choose whether to yield to or resist particular inclinations. Our choices determine what we do and who we are.

* * *

Once we define behavior—any behavior, such as killing oneself or another person, feeling depressed, persecuted, or shy—as a disease or as the symptom of a disease, and accept it and treat it as if it were a disease, we are off to the races. Leading to where? To controlling behavior—our own and that of others—by chemical, physical, and social interventions called "treatments" and by state-sanctioned force. Medicalizing the control of behavior leads inexorably to pharmacracy and the therapeutic state.

Birth Control

In the landmark case of *Griswold v. Connecticut* (1965), the Supreme Court repealed the Connecticut state law prohibiting the sale of contraceptive devices.[3]

The Court did not medicalize the alleged "condition"—not wanting to procreate—as a disease, nor did it call for "legalizing physician-assisted contraception" as a "treatment" for it.

Instead, the right to practice contraception was placed in the hands of the people, where it belongs, not in the hands of physicians, who have no legitimate need for it.

This ruling ought to be our model for laws prohibiting drugs and suicide. It placed the right to a formerly prohibited practice in the hands of the people, where it belongs, not in the hands of physicians, who have no legitimate need for it.

Brain-Mind

"[The Swartz] Foundation operates from the philosophical and *scientific* perspective that properties of the mind—from sensory perception to learning to thinking to consciousness—are a *direct product of the intrinsic physical properties of the brain. The mind is the brain at work.*"[4]

Calling one's prejudice "science" does not make it so. Michael Polanyi, scientist turned philosopher, warned: "The recognition...of the impossibility of understanding living things in terms of physics and chemistry, far from setting limits to our understanding of life, will guide it in the right direction."[5]

Werner Heisenberg, one of the giants of modern physics, stated: "[O]ne will nowadays be less inclined to assume that the concepts of physics, even those of quantum theory, can certainly be applied everywhere in biology or other sciences.[6]

It is naive to believe that attributing mental functions to brain functions is a new idea or that the dominant mechanical model of the moment—today, the computer—"explains" how "the mind works."

The modern scientist's search for the seat of the mind is but a new version of the medieval scholar's search for the seat of the soul. Descartes (1596-1650) located the soul in the pineal gland. When science displaced religion, the mind replaced the soul and people began to look for the seat of the mind. Not surprisingly, they found it in the brain, rediscovering the "discovery" of the great pagan physician.

Hippocrates (460-377 B.C.), the "father of medicine," stated: "And men ought to know that from nothing else but thence [from the brain] come joys, delights, laughter and sports, and sorrows, griefs, despondency, and lamentations.... And by the same organ we become mad and delirious, and fears and terrors assail us."

C

Charlatan

Webster's defines a charlatan as "a pretender to medical knowledge; one making especially noisy or showy pretenses to knowledge or ability." The charlatan's goals are fame and fortune.

Formerly—when patients paid for treatments—the typical physician-charlatan seduced the public by promises of effective treatments. Patients paid him for fake cures.

Today—when insurance companies pay for treatments—the typical physician-charlatan scares the public with warnings about ineffective treatments. Plaintiff's lawyers pay him for fake testimony. (See also *Quackery*)

Child

Children do not ask to be born. Parents create children to give meaning to their lives, not lives to their children.

* * *

A child becomes an adult when he realizes that he has a right not only to be right but also to be wrong.

* * *

In the universe of persons, children rank first as both the most wanted and the most unwanted.

Would-be parents go to extreme lengths to have children, by natural and artificial methods of procreation, adoption, even theft.

At the same time, parents avail themselves of many methods—some legal, some not—to rid themselves of unwanted children. The fetus may be aborted. The infant may be disposed of by adoption or infanticide; the older child, by adoption or confinement in a foster home or orphanage; the adolescent and the adult child, by incarceration in a mental hospital (and, once there, by further destruction of his self by sterilization, electro-shock, lobotomy, or anti-psychotic drugs).

* * *

Our biological existence begins in the womb, our social existence in the family.

Over these beginnings we have no control. Our utter inability to have or exercise our will is, however, short-lived. Soon, we are expected to eat and sleep only at certain times. Next, we are expected to control the functioning of our bladder and bowel, and then all of our musculature.

As social beings, we thus begin our lives with responsibilities: childhood is a period of tutelage during which we are given many responsibilities, but acquire few rights. This important disjunction between responsibilities and rights is repeated, most glaringly, in the institution of slavery, and, less obviously, in the relations between superiors and inferiors in religion, medicine, and the countless paternalistic arrangements through which human beings seek to reinstate the original parent-child relationship.

* * *

The child cannot match the adult in most accomplishments. Hence, we reward him for effort as well as achievement. Yet, the child must learn that what counts in life is not effort but achievement. The child over-rewarded for effort may grow up to seek approval for trying instead of for succeeding. This dooms him to failure. If he succeeds, he succeeds only at trying hard. If he fails, he fails miserably.

* * *

It is difficult for a son to compete with a successful father, but it may be even more difficult to compete with an unsuccessful one.

Many young men find the prospect of their own failure easier to bear than the prospect of being the instruments of their fathers' humiliation.

* * *

Parents ought to teach the child obedience for two very different reasons: to render him submissive to them and to enable him to become independent of them.

Only a self-disciplined person can be obedient; and only such a person can be autonomous.

* * *

Some parents want their children to *have* it better; others want them to *do* better. The former are likely to have incompetent and unhappy children, the latter, competent and happy ones.

* * *

The child wants to grow up because he experiences his life as constrained by authority. Adulthood beckons because he perceives it as a condition of greater liberty.

But what is there in America today that a very poor or a very rich adolescent wants to do but cannot do? Not much: He can *do* drugs, *have* sex, *make* babies, and *get* money (from parents or the state). For such a young person, adulthood means responsibility rather than liberty. It should not surprise us if he chooses to remain an adolescent.

* * *

Juvenile court judges now routinely send children deemed to be "ungovernable" or "in need of supervision" to psychiatrists.

The child correctly views the psychiatrist so imposed on him as his adversary. The psychiatrist insists on viewing himself as the protector of the child's best interests.

The parents who initiate this process, and juvenile court judges who mandate it, also insist on viewing themselves as helping the child—to receive the "treatment" he needs.

If we wanted to hasten the destruction of children injured by parental neglect, it would be difficult to devise a more effective method for doing so.

* * *

In America today, we tend to treat children as adults, and adults as children. The options of children are thus steadily expanded, while those of adults are progressively constricted. The result is unruly children and childish adults.

* * *

In America today, we also tend to act as if there were no bad children, only mentally ill children who need treatment:

> HELP END SCHOOL VIOLENCE: NAMI CALLS FOR ROUTINE SCREENING OF CHILDREN FOR MENTAL ILLNESS—Statement of Jacqueline Shannon, President, Board of Directors, National Alliance for the Mentally Ill, March 13, 2001. (NAMI E-News March 13, 2001 Vol. 01-83)
>
> Violence in America's schools is no longer rare; it's epidemic.... As the mother of a son with schizophrenia, and a former classroom teacher, I earnestly hope the epidemic of school violence forces us to confront the fact that, contrary to some popular misconceptions, children and adolescents do develop *diagnosable and treatable mental illnesses. Early diagnosis, appropriate intervention and treatment can save lives....* Too often, children with mental disorders go undiagnosed.... NAMI and the Center for the Advancement of Children's Mental Health at Columbia University are working hard to introduce a program called DISC—the Diagnostic Interview Schedule for Children to communities around the country.[1]

* * *

Children are biologically immature and hence incapable of learning the socially most desirable kind of sexual habit, namely, heterosexual, genital intercourse. For this reason, and also because children are physically and politically weaker than adults, they ought to be protected from sexual experiences with adults.

At the same time, because children have control over their own sexual self-stimulation and ought to learn to control their bodily functions, they ought not be prevented from engaging in masturbation, in private.

Child Psychiatry

From a conventional point of view, child psychiatry is a medical specialty devoted to the diagnosis, treatment, and prevention of the mental diseases that afflict children.

From a sociological viewpoint, child psychiatry is a secular institution for regulating domestic relations.

From my point of view, it is a form of child abuse.

* * *

Mental diseases supposedly afflicting children are undeniably misbehaviors. The child mental patient is in an even more helpless position than the adult mental patient. This makes child psychiatry a doubly problematic enterprise.

John S. Werry, professor of psychiatry emeritus at the University of Auckland, New Zealand, comes close to admitting this, and more. He writes: "*[M]any children seen in clinics do not have true disorders but problems of living—developmental conflicts with parents, schools or peers....* Poverty, untreatability, chance and the desire to escape punishment, rather than need for medical attention are often the tickets of entry to child psychiatric services. Child psychiatry has persistently avoided debating this issue.[2]

* * *

Child mental illness as child misbehavior:

Oppositional Disorder, 313.81

> The essential feature is a pattern of disobedient, negativistic, and provocative opposition to authority figures.... The oppositional attitude is toward family members, particularly the parents, and towards teachers.[3]

This is the description of a conflict between two persons of unequal power—the superior person defining the inferior person as mentally ill.

* * *

Formerly, parents and psychiatrists tortured sexually active ("self-abusing") children with mechanical restraints.

Today, they torture behaviorally active ("hyperactive") children with chemical restraints (psychoactive drugs).

* * *

When a woman finds having a fetus in her body annoying, she can abort it by taking an abortifacient drug or having a surgical abortion.

When a woman finds having a child in her home annoying, she can abort his persona by having a child psychiatrist give him a chemical straitjacket.

* * *

The manufacture of mad children:

> According to the Surgeon General's Report on Mental Health, one child in five has signs and symptoms of a mental illness or substance abuse disorder,

yet fewer than one in three are receiving appropriate treatment.... The good news is that we can help most children and adolescents who suffer from psychiatric disorders. The tragedy is that so many children still do not receive the comprehensive, individualized treatment they need and deserve.[4]

* * *

The child psychiatrist is one of the most dangerous enemies not only of children, but also of adults who care for the two most precious and vulnerable things in life—children and liberty.

Child psychiatry—like psychiatric slavery, of which it is an important part—cannot be reformed. It must be abolished.

Child Therapy

Child abuse masquerading as "clinical help."

Choice

When is a choice not a choice? Whenever someone claims it is not and someone else believes him.

The actor himself asserts that his choice was not a choice: apologizing for a minor social infraction, a person says, "I am sorry, I was not myself"; if a person kills another, he claims he is not guilty of murder by reason of insanity.

A person other than the actor asserts that the actor's choice was not a choice: a young woman starves herself and her parents claim she is suffering from anorexia nervosa; a person is charged with a crime and his court-appointed attorney claims he is not guilty because his crime was a product of mental illness, not choice.

Cohabiting

For many people, cohabiting architecturally and cohabiting sexually are mutually antagonistic enterprises.

Colonialism, American

In the nineteenth century, the American government protected Indians by giving them their own turf, called a "reservation," and by letting them use alcohol as an antidepressant and violence as recreation.

In the twentieth century, the American government protected blacks by giving them their own turf, called an "inner city," and by letting them use cocaine as an antidepressant and violence as recreation.

Communism

The religious doctrine that only the powerless deserve to be powerful, and only the poor deserve to be rich.

Community

A true community consists of like-minded persons who respect and have a certain amount of affection for one another. Fundamental to such a community is the group's privilege to include some persons and exclude others.

In short, community implies the community's right to discriminate and reject persons from membership, without having to justify their exclusion. Demonizing individuals and groups for rejecting some persons prevents people from accepting and embracing the Other as a member of the human community.

Contemporary communitarians ignore the fundamental incompatibility between a true community and current American law, typically used to compel unlike-minded persons to associate with one another. The communitarians' effort to rebuild community is like a cocktail-party host's effort to turn it into an intimate affair. The war against discrimination has turned modern societies into giant cocktail parties to which everyone is invited, with noise and tumult replacing intimacy and trust.

Conceit

The religious and nationalist zealot says: My faith and my country are the best, blessed by God.

The madman says: I am the best, I am the Savior.

Religion and nationalism transform illegitimate personal conceit into legitimate collective conceit.

Constitution

In 1865, having grown old and senile, the Constitution died. However, its memory survives and serves as an indispensable rhetorical device for speakers and writers pleading their particular versions of liberty and justice.

Control

Control communicates care and devotion to children, condescension and disdain to adults. Herein lies a fundamental dilemma of society: It ought to encourage parents to love and control their children, and politicians to respect their fellow citizens and leave them alone.

We are well on our way to inverting this arrangement: We encourage parents to fake respect for their children and thus justify their failure to control them; and politicians to fake love for their fellow citizens and thus justify their efforts to exercise capricious control over them.

* * *

Formerly, when people sought to control calamitous events by prayer, they attributed problems to the will of spirits or gods. They called that "religion." We call it "animism."

Today, when people seek to control calamitous events by treatment, they attribute problems to diseases. We call that "medical science." I call it "therapeutism."

Cooperation

Cooperation between people requires only mutual respect. It does not require that they agree about matters unrelated to their joint endeavor.

Crime

The adage "Crime does not pay" is false. If it were true, there would be no crime.

* * *

Every American boy does not have a shot at being president. But every American boy can take a shot at the president.

The road to fame is often closed, but the road to infamy is always open.

* * *

Crime is a *performance,* which occurs at a specific time, in a specific place, whereas mental illness is a *proclivity*, illustrated by the term "dangerousness."

Jones is accused of stealing a Chevrolet belonging to Smith. To convict him of the crime, it must be shown that he stole the Chevrolet in question. Showing that he had stolen a Buick a month earlier is irrelevant to the accusation.

Jones is accused of being suicidal. To commit him to a mental hospital, it need not be shown that he has tried to kill himself. Claiming that he spoke about suicide a month earlier is sufficient evidence.

In short, it is possible to prove that a person has not committed a particular act, but it is impossible to prove that he may not commit it.

Crisis

The word "crisis" comes from the Greek for choice or crossroads. Its core meanings are choice, challenge, opportunity, and risk. It is significant that we use the word to mean disaster, catastrophe, emergency, plight, and predicament.

Cui Bono?

Criminals don't need criminologists.

Psychotics don't need psychiatrists.

Criminologists and psychiatrists are needed by individuals and institutions to justify the coercive control of persons categorized as "criminals" and "psychotics."

D

Dangerousness

A psychiatrist lamenting the stigma of mental illness dismisses the view that "People with mental illnesses are dangerous to others" as a false, "stigmatizing belief about mental illness."[1]

If psychiatrists really believe that, why don't they demand the immediate repeal of commitment laws and refuse to hospitalize people against their will?

* * *

U.S. Justice Department, 2002: "67 percent of inmates released from state prisons in 1994 were rearrested for at least one new, serious crime within three years.... The recidivism rate [was] for 41 percent of those rearrested [who] had been imprisoned for homicide, 46 percent for rape, and 51 percent for driving under the influence of drugs or alcohol."[2]

Nevertheless, the principal justification for preventive psychiatric detention (civil commitment) is "dangerousness."

Death

Primitive man does not recognize natural death: he interprets dying of disease as a *type of homicide*, perpetrated by a person or spirit.

Modern man does not recognize voluntary death; he interprets killing oneself as *a disease, an event* caused by neurotransmitters or mental illness.

* * *

Prior to the advent of organ transplantation, we had only one word and meaning for death. Now, we have two: brain death and organismic death.

We use the concept of brain death to justify removing organs for transplantation from live patients and for discontinuing life support, and the concept of organismic death for burying or cremating the corpse.

Brain death is the death of a part of the body only. We do not call brain-dead persons corpses or their bodies "cadavers," and do not let medical students dissect or undertakers bury their bodies.

* * *

The popular phrase, "death with dignity," is misleading. It is not just that people want to die with dignity, but rather that they want live with it. It is because many people live without dignity that they also die without it. Dying, after all, is a part of life, not death.

Deception

What we call "psychosis" is, in large part, self-deception.

The person who refuses to deceive himself will not become psychotic. However, facing the facts of his life, he may decide to kill himself and thus invite others to call him "psychotic."

Decision

The most serious decision we face in life is whether to commit suicide. The second most serious decision is whether to have or not have a child.

Deinstitutionalization

The Emancipation Proclamation did not free a single slave from domination by the white man.

Deinstitutionalization did not free a single institutionalized mental patient from domination by the psychiatrist.

Delusion

Psychiatrists say that the man who claims to be Jesus suffers from a delusion. They do not say that the man who claims the Eucharist is the body and blood of Jesus suffers from a delusion.

We have a choice to assume that the person who asserts a patently false claim believes it to be literally true, uses it as metaphor, or simply lies.

We are free to believe or disbelieve such a claim—to accredit it as religion, or discredit it as psychosis.

In either case, we are free to leave the claimant alone.

If the law requires the psychiatrist to persecute the psychotic and the psychiatrist believes that is wrong, he could quit his job. (See also *Mental Illness*)

Demagogue

Formerly, the demagogue ruled by appealing to the need to protect the nation from saboteurs and subversives. Today, he rules by appealing to the need to protect "kids" from drugs and pornography.

Depression

If your body is injured, you feel pain. If your mind is injured, you feel depressed.

* * *

Drug treatment of depression: treating a nondisease with a nonmedicine.[3] (See also *Mental Illness*)

Desire

People have diverse, mutually incompatible desires—for liberty and equality, adventure and security, autonomy and intimacy.

The satisfaction of one member of such a pair intensifies the desire for its opposite, which it frustrates. This is one of the reasons why it is foolish to identify any particular human desire with a socially shared Common Good or General Welfare.

Diagnosis

Diagnoses are not diseases.
Diagnoses are names, human fabrications.
Diseases are phenomena, facts of nature.

* * *

Medical diagnoses are the names physicians give to the body parts whose malfunctioning they have identified. Psychiatric diagnoses are the names psychiatrists give to the persons whose misbehavior they have judged.

* * *

The diagnosis of bodily illness justifies a physician to admit to a hospital a patient who wants to be admitted to a hospital.

The diagnosis of mental illness justifies a judge to forcibly "hospitalize" a sex offender who has served his prison sentence.

* * *

Psychiatric diagnoses are dangerously misleading not only because their Greco-Latin names falsely imply that they are bona fide diseases, but also because their social consequences are likely to be injurious to the patient's best interests, as he sees them.

The epistemological validity of a psychiatric diagnosis is separate and distinct from its practical consequence.

If psychiatric diagnoses of mental illnesses were private communications between doctor and patient—which the doctor is as duty-bound to keep confidential as the priest is duty-bound to keep confidential his diagnosis of the penitent's sins—psychiatric diagnoses would still be medically erroneous, but they would be morally unobjectionable.

* * *

Historian David Levering Lewis's characterization of racial lynching is equally valid for psychiatric lynching:

> Lynching was race relations by means of a rope, a sanguinary pageant reenacted by community leaders for whom the untruthfulness of accusations was not merely irrelevant but even an essential element in what was but the everlasting apotheosis of white supremacy.[4]

Mutatis mutandis:

> Psychiatry is lynching by means of a diagnosis, a sanguinary pageant reenacted by psychiatric leaders for whom the untruthfulness of the "patient's illness" is not merely irrelevant but even an essential element in what is but the everlasting apotheosis of psychiatric supremacy.

Dignity

A dignified relationship between persons requires only mutual respect.

Persons of unequal position and power often treat one another with dignity, whereas equals often treat one another in undignified ways.

Discipline

Parents, grandparents, teachers, ministers, and neighbors had, but no longer have, authority to discipline children. Their authority has been pooled and delegated to mental health professionals and psychiatric drugs.

Formerly, adults with a meaningful relationship to the child disciplined him. Now, we look to strangers and drugs to do the job.

Disease

According to Virchow's definition, disease is an objective phenomenon—the patho-anatomical or pathophysiological alteration of the body. At the beginning of the twentieth century, the category called "disease" was expanded to include mental illnesses as diseases on a par with bodily diseases.

According to Christian definition, marriage is a formally recognized social institution: the legal and sexual union of a man and a woman. At the end of the twentieth century (in some Western countries), the category called "marriage" was expanded to include homosexual marriages as legal unions on a par with heterosexual unions.

There is nothing mysterious about such category-creep. The important thing to keep in mind is that it is not based on, and has nothing to do with, new scientific discoveries or knowledge. Instead, it is based on, and is motivated by, ideological, economic, legal, moral, and political interests.

* * *

In the wake of scientific advances in the eighteenth and nineteenth centuries, medical scientists defined the term "disease," for the purpose of scientific discourse, as predicating a biological system. This is why psychiatry, established as a medical specialty in the nineteenth century, was defined as the study of diseases of the brain.

Using the term "mental disease"—as an entity distinct and separate from brain disease—constitutes an expansion of the definition of the term "disease." Such conceptual and definitional expansion is not confined to medicine.

Formerly, the term "marriage" meant the legal union, in a social institution so called, of a man and a woman. Now the term may be used to refer to the legal union, in matrimony, of two men or two women.

Today, the term bachelor is used to refer to an unmarried man. Tomorrow, it may very well also be used to refer to a gay man married to a lesbian woman.

* * *

We can define disease descriptively, as a phenomenon, or prescriptively, as a strategy.

Descriptively, lung cancer is a disease. Prescriptively, smoking is also a disease, justifying political interference with tobacco use on medical grounds.

Descriptively, the intact human penis of the newborn male is "normal." Prescriptively, it is not, justifying the practice of routine neonatal circumcision on medical grounds.

The same principle justifies abortion (on demand); Ritalin (for restless children in school); and Haldol (for restless old people in nursing homes).

* * *

If the government classifies drug use as *behavior*, then it either cannot regulate the use of "dangerous drugs" or must regulate it as a crime.

If the government classifies the use of "dangerous drugs" as "drug abuse"—a *disease*—then it can regulate it as both a public health problem and as a psychiatric problem.

Ignoring the strategic uses of medical terms enables jurists, physicians, mental health professionals, scientists, and journalists to debate, *ad nauseam*, whether alcoholism, smoking, kleptomania, and this or that unwanted behavior is or is not a disease.

* * *

Disease: 1. Proven bodily lesion. 2. Putative bodily lesion. 3. Distress, disability, disadvantage, dysfunction. 4. An (ostensibly) treatable condition. 5. Irrationality. 6. Irresponsibility. 7. Crime. 8. Any human behavior or characteristic we dislike.

* * *

Demonstrable bodily lesion is the gold standard of medical diagnosis. Without practical convertibility into gold, the value of paper money rests only on faith. Without conceptual convertibility into bodily lesion, the diagnosis of disease rests only on faith. Unbacked by gold, paper money is *fiat* money—the politically irresistible incentive for debauching the currency, called "inflation." Unbacked by lesion, diagnosis is *fiat* disease—the medically irresistible incentive for debauching the concept of disease, called "psychiatry."

* * *

The term "illness" can mean either a disease (lesion) or the state of feeling sick (the sense of being ill or unwell). In the former case, "illness" is synonymous with "disease." In the latter case, "illness" is an abstract noun without material or objective referent. Used this way, there is no difference between saying "I feel ill" and saying "I have an illness." Note, however, that *feeling ill* is analogous to *feeling well*, or *happy*, or *sad*; but that it would be nonsensical to replace these expressions with *I have a wellness*, or *I have a happiness*, or *I have a sadness*.

In ordinary use, illness and disease are interchangeable. We say "l feel sick/ill" when we feel indisposed, because of disease or some other reason. In short, feeling ill may or may not be a good reason for assuming the sick role and seeking medical help.

* * *

Bad habits treated as if they are diseases:

Using alcohol badly: "alcoholism." (Treated with AA programs, Antabuse, and other drugs.)

Using food badly: "anorexia nervosa," "obesity." (The former is treated with electroshock, the latter with intestinal bypass operations.)

Using drugs badly: "addiction," "drug abuse." (Treated with imprisonment and diverse psychiatric tortures.)

Using language badly: "psychosis." (Treated with psychiatric incarceration and anti-psychotic drugs.)

* * *

In the case of bodily illness, the patient pays, or is willing to pay, the doctor to *relieve him* of being bothered by his illness.

In the case of mental illness, the taxpayer pays the psychiatrist to *relieve us* of being bothered by the patient.

* * *

Establishing that X has a bodily illness (e.g. tuberculosis) does not depend on whether we believe that he has such an illness.

Establishing whether X has a mental illness (e.g. schizophrenia) depends heavily on whether we believe that he has such a disease.

Drug

A drug cannot expand consciousness. The only thing a drug can expand is the earnings of the company that makes it.

* * *

The FDA calls certain substances "controlled." But there are no controlled substances; there are only controlled persons.

* * *

Treating addiction to heroin with methadone is like treating addiction to scotch with bourbon.

* * *

The person whose ability to move his muscles is impaired—by injury, illness, or old age—uses a cane or crutch. The person whose ability to live his life is impaired—by ideas, memories, or social circumstances—uses drugs.

As the crutch helps a person to move his limbs better, the drug helps him to live his life better—in each case, "better" being defined by the subject himself.

* * *

If a mentally ill person takes a drug prescribed for him by a physician and claims that it makes him feel better, that proves that mental illness is a real disease, "treatable" with drugs.

If a mentally healthy person takes a drug prohibited for him by legislators and claims that it makes him feel better, that proves that he has become mentally ill, having succumbed to the disease called "substance abuse."

* * *

As long as there is no free-market competition between prescription drugs and illegal drugs—between Prozac and cocaine, Haldol and opium—the benefits of official psychiatric "medications," as experienced and defined by the subjects, will remain unknown and unknowable.

* * *

Drugs are material entities that can act only on other material entities. There is no such thing as a mind-altering drug. A so-called mind-altering drug alters the brain and the behavior of the person who voluntarily ingests or injects it, or into whose body it is forcibly introduced against his will.

If a person voluntarily uses a drug that alters his behavior, then his altered behavior is, *ipso facto*, the behavior he prefers.

If a person is forcibly drugged with a drug that alters his behavior, then his altered behavior is, *ipso facto*, the behavior his captors prefer.

* * *

Tranquilizing drugs—especially when they are introduced into the body of a person or animal by force or fraud—ought to be called "domesticating drugs." Their purpose and function is to make the person's or pet's behavior more comfortable for the person/owner doing the drugging.

Dr. Petra Mertens, a German veterinarian, explained: "The number of cats taking psychiatric drugs has soared over the last ten years." Note that the cats are "taking psychiatric drugs," exactly as children and mental patients forcibly drugged are said to be "taking" drugs.

Why are cats "taking" Prozac? Because they suffer from "obsessive-compulsive disorders similar to those experienced by humans.... Trials of fluoxetine (Prozac) in the U.S. have shown that cats can be treated with the drug like humans.... If a cat will not take the pill, it can be made into a fish-tasting liquid and used as a treat."[5]

Cui bono?

Drug Laws

Drug laws are our dietary laws: Doctors are our rabbis; heroin, our pork; addicts, our unclean persons.

* * *

Debating the medical value of marijuana with American politicians is like debating the nutritional value of pork with Jewish or Islamic clergymen.

Drug prohibition is a ceremonial symbol of the policymaker's authority. The prohibition has nothing to do with the medical validity of the government's claim about the banned substance.

The more "irrational" a prohibition is, the more powerful is its symbolic function legitimizing the authority's compassion and wisdom, and the greater is its appeal to the faithful.

* * *

Giving oneself a controlled substance is a crime. Accepting it from a physician is a treatment.

* * *

Cigarettes and whisky, which are legal products, cannot be advertised on television. Prescription drugs, which, properly speaking, are illegal products, can be.

* * *

A physician who promotes the intravenous use of illegal drugs is like a Catholic priest who promotes adultery. Neither the physician nor the priest can endorse or facilitate such behavior without compromising his basic values.

This is one of the reasons why I oppose needle exchange as "harm reduction," and support the repeal of drug prohibition.

* * *

We regard state monopoly of the press as a characteristic of a totalitarian society, and state monopoly of the pharmacopoeia as a characteristic of a free society.

* * *

We have no "religion policy." Our political system expects the American people to assume a posture of *caveat emptor* toward the purveyors of religions.

We also have no "press policy." Our political system expects the American people to assume a posture of *caveat emptor* toward the purveyors of pictures and words.

Mutatis mutandis, we do not need a "drug policy." We need a political system that expects the American people to assume a posture of *caveat emptor* toward the purveyors of drugs.

* * *

Drug prohibition is unwise social policy, because forbidden fruit tastes sweeter.

One of the easiest ways for a young person to assert his autonomy is by defying arbitrary and hypocritical authority.

* * *

Prescription laws place the American adult in the role of a child: he wants a cookie but cannot get into the cookie jar—the pharmacopeia—without the help of a doctor. The result is that many people go to doctors, especially family physicians, for the sole purpose of obtaining the prescription drug they want.

* * *

The American people consistently vote for politicians who let them buy guns but prohibit them from buying drugs.

I interpret this to mean that we are more afraid of injecting ourselves with a drug than of being shot by an assailant; more afraid of shooting ourselves metaphorically than of someone else literally shooting us; in short, more afraid of ourselves than of criminals.

* * *

The "Jewish problem" was the name the Nazis gave to their persecution of certain people: Jews, Gypsies, homosexuals.

The "drug problem" is the name we give to our persecution of people who use certain drugs: cocaine, heroin, marijuana.

* * *

Prohibiting a drug makes it more toxic, because the illegal seller adulterates it and has no competitors who sell the same product in unadulterated form.

Not prohibiting a drug makes it less toxic, because the law punishes the legal distributor who sells an adulterated drug and because he has competitors who sell the same product in unadulterated form.

* * *

Some people advocate prohibiting heroin, others, that it be given free to addicts. Both recommendations are foolish.

Why should heroin be prohibited when alcohol and cigarettes are not? Why should heroin be dispensed at the taxpayer's expense, but not alcohol and cigarettes?

It is revealing of our propensity for medical meddling that every conceivable measure for solving "the problem"—except one—is now seriously advocated. Repealing anti-drug laws and leaving so-called addicts alone is unthinkable.

* * *

In 1903, if an American president demanded that farmers in foreign countries not grow certain crops, he would have been ridiculed.

Today, if an American president insisted that farmers in foreign countries have the right to grow any crop they want, he would be diagnosed.

* * *

American politicians denounce the right of foreigners to export their traditional drugs, but defend the right of Americans to export not only alcohol and tobacco but also toxic wastes. "Unlike the trade in drugs...dumping poison in poor countries is perfectly legal," explain reporters for *Newsweek.*[6]

* * *

The idea that treating money as a commodity is a moral wrong generated the criminalization of charging interest, called "usury."

The idea that treating drugs as a commodity is a moral wrong generated the criminalization of trading in drugs, called "drug trafficking."

* * *

The "victims" of drug (ab)use are the persons who use illegal drugs, while the victims of the war on drugs are the persons who do not use such drugs.

Herein lies the ultimate immorality and injustice of anti-drug laws: they value protecting people from their own cravings more highly than protecting people from the criminal violence of other people.

* * *

Drug abuse treatment: the state coercing hardworking persons to pay "addicts" for their "disability," and psychiatrists for treating the nonexisting disease called "addiction."

* * *

Ostensibly, drugs such as marijuana are prohibited because their use impairs the social functioning of the user.

This claim is inconsistent with the fact that the authorities—parents, politicians, and physicians—don't know who uses such drugs: they support costly efforts to develop and deploy tests to find illicit users.

If it were true that illicit drugs impair social functioning (a meaningless idea in the absence of specifying drug and dosage), we wouldn't need special tests to identify the users.

* * *

In the United States, the most important social function of the war on drugs is to convert a potentially violent race war into a presumably therapeutic war on drugs. It accomplishes this goal, in part, by providing bread and circuses for uneducated, unemployed, and unwanted urban youths.

* * *

The behavior we call "drug abuse"—and punish by means of both criminal and psychiatric sanctions—is the result of criminalizing and medicalizing what used to be called "sin."

The parable of the Fall may be viewed as the paradigm of a person who ingests a substance Authority has prohibited him from ingesting.

A devout Jew who eats ham violates religious law. A person who murders violates secular law. A diabetic who fails to take insulin violates medical "law."

We are free to manipulate these categories: indeed, we transform sins into crimes, crimes into sins, and both into diseases. Which of these categorizations we accept or reject depends largely on how we wish to deal with the person who exhibits the (problematic) behavior.

* * *

Formerly, in the Age of Faith, people demonstrated their love of God and fellow man by forcibly converting the heathen and extolling religious coercion as holy.

Today, in the Age of Therapy, people demonstrate their love of Health and fellow man by forcibly treating the addict and extolling therapeutic coercion as noble.

The headline of a full-page ad, sponsored by the Partnership for a Drug Free America, in *Newsweek* magazine, exhorts: "Sometimes, the worst thing you can do to a drug user is the only way to help." The ad invites the reader to call the "National Institute on Drug Abuse hotline."[7]

"Addicts would be better off if more of them were arrested and forced to enroll in treatment programs...[this is] the essence of humane therapy," declares Yale University psychiatrist Sally Satel.[8]

"If any one slay with the sword," warns the Bible, "with the sword he must be slain."[9]

The American people may have to learn moral modesty the hard way, by ever more of them becoming the victims of the war on drugs they so enthusiastically wage.

* * *

Voltaire is said to have declared: "I disapprove of what you say, but I will defend to the death your right to say it."[10]

No prominent literary person or social critic says today: "I disapprove of what drug you take, but I will defend to the death your right to take it."

It seems to me that the right to take things is more elementary than the right to say things, because taking things is less likely to harm others than saying them.

In a free society, it is none of the government's business what idea a man puts into his head; it should also be none of its business what drug he puts into his body.

* * *

A hundred years ago, a person could legally purchase—in the free market, for a small sum—all the pure and safe opium he wanted.

Today, he can illegally purchase—in the black market, for a large sum—a small amount of impure and unsafe opiates.

This is where the anticapitalist mentality combined with faith in pharmacracy has brought us.

* * *

Before 1914, a person could buy and use any drug because he *wanted* to. He did not have to prove to anyone that he *needed* it.

Today, a person can still buy and use a cane or crutch if he *wants* to. He does not have to prove to anyone that he *needs* it. But he cannot buy a prescription drug because he wants it. Instead, he must first prove to a physician that he needs a particular drug. Even then he may not be able to obtain the desired drug because the physician, too, has to demonstrate to the authorities, who sit in judgment on him, that he *needs* to prescribe the "controlled substance."

* * *

The Soviet government censored the press, which led to the creation of a *samizdat* (underground) press. American presidents interpreted that as evidence of the economic and moral superiority of the free market over the command economy.

The American government censors drugs, which led to the creation of a *samizdat* (underground) pharmacopoeia. American presidents interpret this as evidence of the subversion of the free market by "drug lords" and "narcoterrorists."

* * *

The more zealously we transform the drug market from being based on wants ("I want X, am willing to pay for X, hence can buy X") to being based on needs ("I need X, am willing to beg for it from a physician, hence am entitled to receive it free from the state"), the more stupidly and swiftly we march down the road to therapeutic serfdom.

* * *

Vainly, we look to medicine for an understanding of our drug problem. We do so because medicine has replaced religion as the socially accredited method for burying our collective head in the sand. More than a century ago, Samuel Butler wrote:

> No matter how many laws they [the Erewhonians] passed increasing the severity of punishments inflicted on those who ate meat in secret, the people found means of setting them aside as fast as they were made...[and] when they were on the point of being repealed some national disaster or the preaching of some fanatic would reawaken the conscience of the nation, and people were imprisoned by the thousands for illicitly selling and buying animal food.[11]

* * *

The Romans believed that in wine there is truth (*in vino veritas*): Under the influence of alcohol, people often say and do things they would otherwise not say or do.

We believe that in wine there is lunacy: Under the influence of alcohol people often say and do things that are supposedly non-volitional. Such behavior is attributed to ("caused by") the drug.

The Romans considered voluntary intoxication an aggravating condition and punished the actor for crimes committed when under the influence of alcohol more severely than crimes committed when not under the influence of alcohol.

We consider voluntary intoxication an excusing condition and punish the actor for crimes committed when under the influence of alcohol less severely than crimes committed when not under the influence of alcohol. (Motor vehicle violations while under the influence of alcohol are an exception.)

Is this an advance or retrogression in understanding the nature of man, the connection between drugs and behavior, and the proper function of the law?

* * *

Vowing to protect people from "dangerous drugs," politicians wage war on the soil of foreign nations, trying to prevent peasants from growing their traditional crops.

No one needs the government to protect him from "dangerous drugs." Everyone can easily protect himself by not buying or using the stigmatized drug.

* * *

People ingest, inhale, and inject drugs for many reasons other than treating a disease, for example: to feel better; change one's consciousness; facilitate conviviality; celebrate a religious or social occasion; make oneself alert or sleepy, fertile or infertile; enhance one's endurance, athletic performance, or sexual prowess; improve or otherwise change one's appearance.

It makes no more sense to make the use of certain drugs, *regardless of why a person wants it*, contingent on medical approval than it would to make the use of dieting, *regardless of why a person wants it*, contingent on medical approval.

* * *

We have been waging a War on Drugs for almost eighty years. Its obvious results are the destruction of the mechanisms people have used for millennia to protect themselves from dangerous drugs, such as self-discipline and *caveat emptor*, rampant drug abuse, "no-fault mental illnesses," victimology, and the punishing of one or both parties to contractual relations between consenting adults.

Drug Education

The war on drugs: Just say no to drugs the government deems bad for you.

The war on mental illness: Just say yes to drugs the government deems good for you.

* * *

Public schools engage in an activity they call "drug education."

Properly speaking, education is the imparting of accurate information. Drug education is fashionable anti-drug propaganda.

* * *

Approximately 10 percent of American physicians are said to "abuse drugs." Physicians receive enough "drug education" to enable them to understand the action of drugs. Such knowledge is morally indifferent or neutral. A person may use pharmacological information to help or harm himself or others, to obey or disobey custom and law.

E

Economics

In the pre-industrial world, the manual labor of members of the lower classes supported the idle members of the upper classes. The hereditary rich were then believed to have a morally justified claim on the labor of the productive poor.

In the post-industrial world, the intellectual labor of members of the upper and middle classes supports the idle members of the lower classes. The hereditary poor are now believed to have a morally justified claim on the labor of the productive rich.

The entitlements of feudal lords have been transformed into the entitlements of the urban underclass.

* * *

The pioneer economists were moral philosophers and political reformers. The modern economists borrowed the methods and prestige of mathematics and defined economics as a science. In 1968, the Nobel Awards Committee authenticated economics as a science by establishing, with the help of the Bank of Sweden, a Nobel Prize in Economic Sciences.

The pioneer mad-doctors were apothecaries and clergymen. In the nineteenth century, they borrowed the methods and prestige of medicine and defined psychiatry as a medical science. In 1949, the Nobel Awards Committee authenticated psychiatry as a science by awarding the Nobel Prize in Medicine to the Portuguese neurosurgeon Egas Moniz.

* * *

In 1974, Gunnar Myrdal—famous Swedish socialist economist who shared the Nobel Prize in Economic Science with Friedrich Hayek—declared that "the economics prize should be removed because it had been given to such reactionaries as [Milton] Friedman and Hayek."[1]

In 1949, the Nobel Prize in Medicine was awarded to the Portuguese neurosurgeon Egas Moniz for lobotomy as a treatment for "schizophrenia." Yet, no winner of the Nobel Prize for medicine has called for the abolition of the award on that account.

Neither Myrdal nor Moniz was a scientist: neither economics nor psychiatry is a science.

* * *

Modern libertarian economists have hijacked the idea of liberty: they have made freedom appear to be a by-product of the free market. This is a fallacy. Economic growth and material prosperity neither guarantee freedom nor are a measure of it.

Historically, the idea of freedom rests on a moral and philosophical basis. Montesquieu, Voltaire, and Zola in France; Smith, Mill, and Acton in England; Franklin, Jefferson, and Paine in America—none was an economist or based the case for liberty on economic arguments.

I am not gainsaying the crucial importance for individual liberty of the right to property and a rule of law protecting that right. I am merely saying that liberty is not the sole "possession" of free-market economists.

Education

Every act of conscious learning requires the willingness to suffer an injury to one's self-esteem. That is why young children, before they are aware of their own self-importance, learn so easily; and why older persons, especially if vain or important, cannot learn at all.

* * *

Chinese Proverb: "He who asks a question is a fool for a minute; he who does not remains a fool forever."

* * *

Compulsory education is the chink in the armor of American capitalism. We are expected to value initiative and contract, but base our educational system on conformity and compulsion.

* * *

"The more corrupt the state, the more laws." (Tacitus, 56-115)
The more corrupt the education, the more credentials.

Electroshock

A patient with cancer says: "If I had refused my surgeon's suggestion that I have my tumor removed, the cancer would have killed me."

A patient with depression says: "If my psychiatrist had let me refuse the electroshock treatment he recommended, I would have killed myself."

The difference between those two sentences sums up the difference between bodily illness and mental illness.

Empiricist

Empiricists verify and falsify observations. Moralists legitimize or delegitimize claims.

Entitlements

In an aristocracy, the nobleman was entitled, by virtue of his social status, to special privileges, in particular, to the other's labor.

In a pharmacracy, the authenticated victim is entitled, by virtue of his social status, to special privileges, in particular, to the other's capital.

Equivalence

The rule of algebraic equivalence: If a=b, then b=a.

If all mental disease is brain disease, then all brain disease is mental disease.

Clearly, this is not true.

The patient suffering from a mental disease, such as schizophrenia, displays no neurological symptoms, yet is said to have a brain disease.

The patient suffering from a brain disease, such as a stroke, displays mental symptoms, but is not said to have a mental disease.

Error

"It is the error alone which needs the support of government. Truth can stand by itself," said Thomas Jefferson.[2]

Because truth can stand by itself, it does not need the support of government.

Because error cannot stand by itself, it needs the support of government. It receives the support of the government because it is useful for supporting the government.

Ethics

To forgive all is to demand all.

* * *

The safest sin: envy, which is easily disguised as enthusiasm for equality.

The most dangerous virtue: tolerance, which is easily construed as sympathy for subversion.

* * *

Bioethics: A front for medical statism.

Bioethicist: Apologist for pharmacracy and the therapeutic state.

* * *

For 200 years, ethicists have generated apologetics for psychiatry, obstructing the development of a moral critique of its inhumane practices. Now, medical ethicists do the same for pharmacracy and its inhumane practices.

* * *

Practicing ethicists either ratify or criticize prevailing mores: medical ethics must be either a celebration or a criticism of prevailing medical practices.

Medical institutions cannot be expected to hire and pay individuals to systematically criticize the practices of their professional staff: the establishment of departments of medical ethics in hospitals and medical schools means that professional medical ethicists are likely to devote themselves to opposing the development of a genuine medical ethics, much as psychiatric ethicists have devoted themselves to opposing the development of a genuine moral critique of psychiatry.

* * *

A glossary:

Bad: Obsolete; superseded by insane, mentally ill, sick.

Good: Obsolete; superseded by sane, mentally healthy, healthy.

Ethics: Obsolete; superseded by the diagnosis and treatment of disease.

* * *

The liberal-scientific ethic: if it's bad for you, it should be prohibited; if it's good for you, it should be required.

* * *

The therapeutic ethic: convict and punish the innocent, and call it mental hospitalization; diagnose and excuse the guilty, and call it the insanity defense.

* * *

The principle of tyranny: anyone not for me is against me. The principle of tolerance: anyone not against me is for me.

* * *

The three principal rules of conduct:

1. The Golden Rule: Do unto others as you want them to do unto you.

2. The Rule of Respect: Do unto others as they want you to do unto them.

3. The Rule of Paternalism: Do unto others as you in your superior wisdom know ought to be done unto them in their own best interests.

* * *

Rules of conduct according to the ethics of autonomy:

- Criticize the oppressor, but do not humiliate him.

- Defend the oppressed, but do not glamorize him.

- Respect everyone, regardless of merit or position.

- Bestow admiration and love because it is deserved, not because you need others to protect and love you.

- Know your enemies; avoid them, if you can; intimidate them if you can't; subdue them, if you must.

- Honor your friends; be loyal to them, if you can; warn them, if you can't.

* * *

"Nobody may compel me to be happy in his own way," said Kant. "Paternalism is the greatest despotism imaginable."[3]

I agree. But imagine what the world would be like if the majority of people believed this and acted accordingly.

* * *

In 1987, historian Barbara Tuchman lamented: "It does seem that the knowledge of the difference between right and wrong is absent from our society, as if it had floated away on a shadowy night after the last World War. So remote is the concept that even to speak of right and wrong marks one to the younger generation as old-fashioned, reactionary, and out of touch."[4]

Ironically, Tuchman supported the mental health movement and was a prominent practitioner of the sinister art of psychohistory. Forty years ago I warned against this danger, citing the program for modern psychiatry outlined by Brock Chisholm at the end of World War II.[5]

During the war, Chisholm was director-general of medical services in the Canadian army. After it, he became the first director of the United Nation's World Health Organization. In 1946, he wrote: "The reinterpretation and eventual eradication of the concept of right and wrong...are the belated objectives of all effective psychotherapy. If the race is to be freed from its crippling burden of good and evil, it must be the psychiatrists who take the original responsibility. This is a challenge which must be met."[6]

Psychiatrists have met the challenge and, aided and abetted by intellectuals, journalists, clergymen, and jurists, helped to destroy the difference between right and wrong and replace it with the difference between mentally healthy and mentally ill. (See also *Medical Ethics*)

* * *

Excluding the Other

The fundamental principle of all social organization is the division of people into two groups: Us versus Them.

Chosen people / Rejected people
Saved / Damned
Faithful / Heretic
God-fearing / Atheist
Master / Slave
White / Black
Native / Foreigner
Civilized / Savage
Literate / Illiterate
Educated / Uneducated
Professional / Lay
Rich / Poor
Healthy / Sick
Sane / Insane
Rational / Irrational
Competent / Incompetent

Excuses

Formerly, people believed in the devil and in contracts, exemplified by the Pact with the Devil.

Now, people believe in neither, exemplified by insolvency and insanity as excuses from contractual obligations.

Expectation

We expect teenagers to be able to control computers but be unable to control their appetites for drugs and sex, and they often fulfill our expectations.

Explanation

In the nineteenth century, the false explanation called "ether" obstructed advances in cosmology, and the false explanation called "spontaneous generation" obstructed advances in biology. Today, the false explanation called "mental illness" obstructs advances in psychology, psychiatry, criminology, and drug policy.

Externalities

Every act has consequences in addition to those intended by the actor. Economists call these effects "externalities."

Although drug (ab)use may adversely affect the user's family, its main victim, if any, is the drug user.

In contrast, drug prohibition adversely affects every member of society, infringing on his liberty and reducing his opportunity for self-disciplined behavior. The negative externalities of drug prohibition thus far exceed those of a free market in drugs.

F

Family

There are two kinds of parental love: one is expressed by the gentle but firm expectation that the child "can do it," the other, by the vague and vacuous declaration of an unconditional acceptance bordering on approval.

Expectation of good behavior encourages competence and implies respect for the child. Unconditional acceptance discourages competence and implies disrespect for him.

* * *

Prolonged, unrelieved association between children and parents is likely to prove irritating to one or both parties. Out of this elementary fact psychiatrists fashion elaborate theories about why and how parents drive their children crazy and vice versa. ("Insanity is hereditary. Parents get it from their children.")

Although everyone needs human contact, both physical and spiritual, too much contact engenders feelings of antagonism toward those who infringe on one's life-space. This is why children often experience parental protection not as love but as deprivation of independence.

Furor

Furor therapeuticus. A characteristic of the nineteenth-century physician: few effective treatments, many cures.

Furor diagnosticus. A characteristic of the twentieth-century psychiatrist: few patients with real diseases, many diagnoses.

G

Gambling

Most people experience life as a process of getting nothing for something: they work long hours, pay taxes, care for their families, and end their lives in sickness and poverty.

The enchantment of gambling lies in reversing—or at least the possibility of reversing—this process: getting something for nothing.

* * *

The excitement and mystery of gambling lies in a neglected characteristic of the experience—namely, the subjective sense of being in complete control of one's decisions. This sense of subjective control is independent of one's objective chances of winning or losing.

Although gambling is seemingly social, it is in fact solitary: physically, the gambler is in the presence of others; psychologically, he is alone, uninfluenced by anyone. For the moment, he is Walter Mitty, exhilarated by the experience of autonomous decision-making.

This, combined with the hope of winning, is why gambling is the biggest legal business in America.

* * *

Daniel Goleman, Ph.D., psychologist and *New York Times* writer:

> The psychological forces that propel so many chronic gamblers to ruin marriages, lose jobs, and even turn to crime may spring from a biological need...pathological gamblers suffer from an addiction like alcoholism...gamblers had lower levels than usual of the brain chemicals that regulate arousal…they may engage in activities like gambling to increase their levels of these chemicals in the noradrenergic system, which secretes them.[1]

I prefer my definition of the pathological gambler as a gambler who loses money, not his wife.

And I still think that people gamble because they enjoy it and hope to win, not because they want to increase the levels of "chemicals in the noradrenergic system" of their bodies.

* * *

Amin Daghestani, professor of psychiatry at Loyola University in Chicago:

> Compulsive gambling is a damaging disease for an estimated nine million Americans. Physicians everywhere must recognize this problem as a treatable, medical condition.[2]

Gender

The most basic, albeit involuntary, "contract" with our fellow man is that our gender self-identification is consistent with our chromosomally defined sexual identity. Departure from this convention disorients and disorders social relations: cross-dressing, homosexuality, and transsexualism, in that order, disrupt the subject's relations to his parent, spouse, child, friend, and society. This is why each of these behaviors has been prohibited and punished by religion, law, and psychiatry.

The term "involuntary contract" is, of course, a self-contradiction. Because the sexual identity contract is involuntary, some persons feel—for complex reasons—entitled to reject it as a legitimate limitation of their "natural liberty." Society exacts a high price for this form of self-assertion. (See also *Sex*)

Genetics

A report in the *British Medical Journal* informs us that "all humans are 99.99% genetically identical and there is no gene for race."[3]

It is reassuring, however, that there is a gene for schizophrenia.

* * *

In the twentieth century, politicians used genetics to justify medical murder. In the twenty-first century, they use it to justify medical mendacity.

Genius

The term "genius" comes from the Latin root meaning "to generate" or "beget." In the classical world, the term denoted a tutelary god or controlling spirit allotted to each person at birth: genius was a universal human quality, the very opposite of something exceptional.

The modern idea of genius as exceptional talent and/or madness is an eighteenth-century invention. We use one aspect of genius to "explain" the exceptionally meritorious behavior of a person guided by good "voices" ("artistic inspiration"), and another aspect of it to "explain" the exceptionally deplorable behavior of a person guided by bad "voices" ("command hallucinations").

Getting Along

"To get along, you go along," teaches the proverb. That's easy, but it will cost you your integrity.

If you want to preserve your integrity, you must learn the secret of getting along without going along, which requires, above all else, being civil and respectful toward people with whom you want to get along but not go along.

God

The grand justifier and legitimizer; the all-purpose, irrefutable justification, especially for hating and killing and feeling good about it.

* * *

The drug that annuls the conscience.

* * *

Prayer is a manifestation of the megalomania of the helpless: the child, the sick, the person in desperate danger. ("There are no atheists in the foxhole.")

* * *

For the theist, God is the sum of all the possibilities he can imagine. For the atheist, he is the sum of all the impossibilities he can imagine.

H

Habit

Mental illnesses resemble habits, not diseases. A typical mental illness—say, schizophrenia—is a continuation of the person's habits. That is why patients with schizophrenia, who don't want to give up their habits, refuse treatment.

Bodily illnesses resemble power outages, not habits. A typical bodily illness—say, pneumonia—is a disruption of the person's habits. That is why patients with pneumonia, who want to resume their habits, accept treatment.

Hallucination (see Mental Illness)

Hatred

Formerly, debasing the Other by calling him a "nigger" was considered politically correct: the speaker was viewed as a protector of the race or nation from those bent on defiling it.

Today, debasing the Other by calling him "sick" is considered politically correct: the speaker is viewed as a protector of the debased person's best mental health interests and of the nation from a danger to public health.

Replacing the former rhetoric by the latter is considered moral progress.

Health Care

Most people accept that rich and poor do not eat the same kinds of food, wear the same kinds of clothes, live in the same kinds of homes, or have the same kinds of vacations. But most people believe that rich and poor ought to have access to—and receive—the same kinds of health care services. Such is the genius of the modern health care policymaker.

* * *

People have always longed for "universal health care" and politicians always supplied them with this service—or, more precisely, with a policy that the masses accepted as such a service. In the Middle Ages, it was called Catholicism. In the twentieth century, it was called Communism. In the twenty-first century, we call it Universal Health Insurance.

* * *

Dr. Nikolai Alexandrovich Semashko, Lenin's associate and the first head of the Commissariat of Health of the USSR:

> The perspective of communist medicine...[is] the taking over by the state of the responsibility of providing for everyone, at his earliest need, a free and well-qualified medical treatment. Only then will disappear...all private hospitals and all commercial private practice.[1]

* * *

Medicare pays for Viagra, not for food.

Coitus is not essential for health, calories are.

This inconsistency illustrates that it is not possible to demarcate goods and services necessary for health, (that ought to be) provided by the state, from those not necessary for it, provided by the market.

Health Insurance

What we euphemistically call "health insurance" violates the basic economic premise of insurance—protecting people from serious economic losses due to *injurious happenings*, not defraying the expense of existential gains secured by engaging in enjoyable actions.

It makes economic sense to insure a person against the loss of his house due to fire or the loss of his health due to leukemia; it makes legal sense that faking an accident or setting a fire to collect insurance are crimes.

It defies economic sense to "insure" a person for the cost of enjoying sexual intercourse aided with Viagra or avoiding the pain of unwanted pregnancy with the aid of birth control pills; it makes no sense for health insurance companies to pay for smoking cessation, alcoholism "treatment," and similar measures: these "conditions" are the results of voluntary choices in the pursuit of pleasure that can be "cured" by voluntary abstinence, without "medical" aids.

* * *

The typical contractor of homeowner's insurance is the homeowner. He buys insurance to protect himself from costly loss to his house caused by events outside his control, such as fire, not to defray the recurring expense of maintaining it. The ideal outcome for both the buyer and the seller of home and automobile insurance is for the policyholder to never make use of his policy.

The typical contractor of health insurance is not the insured person but his employer. Neither party is free to negotiate the terms of the policy. The employee cannot bargain for a lower premium in exchange for a deductible or for declining coverage for alcoholism or schizophrenia. The employer, who pays part or most of the cost of insurance, is not free to decline coverage for state-mandated medical services.

Everyone knows but no one admits that health insurance is not true insurance. Indeed, Americans now view their health insurance as an open-ended entitlement for reimbursement for virtually any expense that may be categorized as "health care," such as the cost of birth control pills or Viagra.

Health Maintenance Organization

Health Maintenance Organization (HMO): An institution authorized to deny insurance payment to physicians for medical services they deem essential for patients—not to mention what patients deem essential for their own health.

"Hearing Voices"

Term used by psychiatric patients to identify their disavowed thoughts, and by psychiatrists to identify the patients as victims of brain diseases requiring involuntary hospitalization and treatment.

Help

Being helped to do what we can do for ourselves is likely to demean us, whether we know it or not.

The weaker the person helped—the child, the poor, the sick—the more unnecessary help demeans him.

Hospital

Prior to World War II, patients spent long periods in hospitals and received lots of treatment. Now, they spend brief periods in hospitals and receive much less treatment.

The moral: The quantity of medical treatment is inversely proportional to its effectiveness.

Human Beings

Big people make big mistakes.

* * *

People who feel harried regret the past, fear the future, and have no time to live in the present.

Humanity

There is a lot of inhumanity in humanity.

Hypnosis

Two people lying to each other, each pretending to believe both his own and his partner's lies.

* * *

Hypnotic influence is often viewed as an especially powerful form of suggestion, and being "hypnotizable" as being particularly "suggestible."

We call people soaking up the message of a successful demagogue "suggestible." However, we do not call people influenced by the truth "suggestible"; we call them "reasonable."

I regard this as evidence that calling a person "suggestible" or "hypnotizable" implies that he willingly, indeed eagerly, accepts being lied to.

* * *

Hypnosis stands in the same relation to sleep as a person imagining that he is wealthy stands to his being wealthy.

* * *

Webster's defines hypnosis as "a state that resembles normal sleep but differs in being induced by the suggestions and operations of a hypnotizer..."

That definition is a symptom of our civilization's having replaced religious magic with psychiatric magic, religious delusions with psychiatric delusions.

Hypocrisy

Hypocrisy is the oil that lubricates the engine of society. That, however, does not justify over-lubricating it.

I

Identity

Our private, subjective identity is not the same as our public, social identity. William James called social identity the Social Self and defined it as "the recognition which he [a man] gets from his mates."[1]

A person's past—his mother tongue, the culture and religion into which he was born, and so forth—is a part of him, but he need not be a part of it.

Law and society may impose a self on him, but he is who he thinks he is, provided he can free himself of the identities imposed on him by others.

Illness

New York Times: "No one in America, regardless of socially constructed race, should be getting sick," say scientists.[2]

Race is socially constructed. Mental illness is not: it is a genetic disease. (See also *Disease*)

* * *

Incontinence

We call the person who cannot control his bladder "incontinent of urine."

We don't, but ought to, call a person who cannot control himself "incontinent of self." Instead we call him "mentally ill," suffering from bipolar illness or schizophrenia.

Independence

Independence is the prize for making it in life. Dependence is the consolation prize for not making it.

Infanticide

Committed by the mother: postnatal birth control; a symptom of mental illness—postpartum depression—caused by a "chemical imbalance in the brain."

Committed by a stranger: murder.

The same is true for puericide, or killing a child: if committed by the mother, it is a symptom of postpartum depression; if by a stranger, it is murder.

Inflation

Credit expansion stimulates consumerism by encouraging people to buy things they don't need, in the vain hope that it will make them happy.

Diagnostic expansion stimulates therapeutism by encouraging people to seek treatments they don't need, in the vain hope that it will make them healthy.

Injury

Roman philosopher Marcus Aurelius (121-180) counseled, "Reject your sense of injury, and the injury itself disappears."[3]

American lawyers recommend, "Treasure your sense of injury, and we'll turn it into a treasure for you (and us)."

Jesse Jackson, Binjamin Wilkomirski, and their like, urge, "Treasure your sense of injury (genuine or counterfeit), and people will revere you as if you made the world a better place."

Insanity

Jurists, lawyers, philosophers, and mental health professionals often assert that "insanity" is a purely legal term. That claim is a brazen falsehood.

"Heresy" is a purely religious term. No medical or psychological expert is allowed to testify, under oath, that a defendant is a heretic.

If "insanity" were a purely legal term, no medical or psychological expert would be allowed to testify, under oath, that a defendant is insane. (See also *Mental Illness*, *Irrationality*)

Insanity Defense

1. A tactic for legitimizing psychiatry as a bona fide medical specialty and the psychiatrist as a medical expert on insanity/mental illness as a cause of crime.

2. A tactic for classifying/legitimizing the defendant as the type of murderer on whom the law cannot legitimately impose a death penalty.

3. A tactic for classifying/legitimizing the defendant as the type of criminal whose control should be diverted from the criminal justice system to the mental health system.

4. A sacred psychiatric ritual, often confused with the scientific search for the cause of a specific crime.

5. A ceremonial affirmation of the modern legal system's moral grandeur, imposing punishment only on persons responsible for lawless acts committed with free will, and providing "treatment" for persons not responsible for lawless acts committed because of insanity.

* * *

The insanity defense did not arise and does not function as a protection for the defendant. Daniel McNaghten was ready to die for his crime. John Hinckley wanted to die for it.

The insanity defense arose and functions as a protection for the jury and society from having to impose the death penalty on the defendant. Like all "psychiatric help" imposed on individuals against their will, the insanity defense and insanity disposition make the coercers feel good about themselves.

* * *

There is a cynical symmetry between the insanity plea and the insanity disposition.

The criminal (often) says: "My illegal act was not motivated by an intention to do harm or break the law; it was caused by my insanity. (I lacked *mens rea*.)"

The legal-psychiatric system answers: "Our incarcerating you is not motivated by an intention to punish you; it is caused by our obligation to treat your mental illness. (It is a civil, not a criminal, sanction.)

* * *

The French proverb warns: *Qui s'excuse, s'accuse* (He who excuses himself, accuses himself). Similarly, he whom we excuse, we accuse.

The insanity defense is essential for the integrity of psychiatry: it formally recognizes the psychiatrist as a lawful and legitimate excuser, and accuser.

Failure to condemn the insanity defense is fatal for the integrity of mental patient liberation movements: ex-mental patients loudly condemn psychiatric coercions (involuntary mental hospitalization), but quietly endorse psychiatric excuses (the insanity defense).

* * *

The insanity defense and the insanity verdict are joined in holy matrimony in the insanity trial. The defendant claims the fictitious condition/illness "insanity" as an excuse for what he did to his victim. The court claims the same fictitious condition/illness as a justification for what it does to the defendant.

* * *

Formerly, Americans charged with murder were considered innocent until proven guilty; now they are considered insane until proven sane.

* * *

When a woman systematically drowns her five children, everyone speculates about her motives and attributes her act to mental illness. Holding her responsible for her act is considered callous as well as unscientific ("denying the reality of mental illness").

When a man systematically rapes five women, no one speculates about his motives or attributes his act to mental illness. Everyone correctly assumes that the rapist rapes because that is what he wants to do. The absurdity of the idea of "involuntary rape"—of the act being due to mental illness, a "chemical imbalance" in the actor's brain—is self-evident.

Yet, rape is a type of sexual behavior. We know that sexual behavior is mediated by chemicals. We have no similar knowledge about chemicals mediating murderous behavior.

Regardless of our knowledge of the chemical correlates of sexual behavior, we refrain from attributing sexual acts to chemicals and do not excuse rape as caused by mental illness (sex hormones disequilibrating the brain).

We recognize that, precisely because chemicals in our bodies (and other factors) inflame our sexual desires, we must learn to control our sexual behavior and ought to be held responsible for committing illegal sexual acts.

* * *

Liberals and psychiatrists say that the two main causes of crime are mental illness and poverty.

We believe that insanity causes crime, accept insanity as an excusing condition, recognize a special defense (the "insanity defense"), and ask psychiatrists to explain to juries whether a particular case of murder was due to insanity or to free will.

If we truly believe that poverty causes crime, we must accept poverty as an excusing condition, recognize a special defense (the "poverty defense"), and ask economists to explain to juries whether a particular case of theft was due to poverty or free will.

* * *

Gastroenterologists cannot ascertain what was in another person's stomach days, weeks, or months ago. But psychiatrists testify under oath about what was in another person's mind days, weeks, months, or even years ago.

* * *

At the Nuremberg trial of the Nazi war criminals, prosecutor Sir Hartley Shawcross declared: "Crimes do not cease to be criminal because they have a political motive."[4]

At the trial of Oliver North, the prosecutor declared: "When an individual is asked a question by Congress, there are only two legitimate responses: the individual may decline to answer the question, or answer it honestly. He cannot with impunity...answer with a falsehood.... [North's] alleged motivation for lying is irrelevant to the charges against him."[5]

Mutatis mutandis, I maintain that a person who believes he should kill someone—say, because he "hears voices" ordering him to do so—has only two legitimate choices: he can control himself and not kill another person, or he can kill himself.

The alleged motivation for murder—say, obeying God's command to kill one's children because they are possessed by the devil—ought not to be a claim admissible in court.

* * *

The popular belief that "society is responsible for crime, and criminals are not responsible for crime," sociologist Arnold W. Green points out, amounts to the view that "only those members of society who do not commit a crime can be held responsible for crime. Nonsense this obvious can be circumvented only by conjuring up society as devil, as evil apart from people and what they do."[6]

Insanity as evil apart from what a specific, allegedly insane person does is an even more obvious nonsense; it is also even more appealing, because it makes illness rather than society the culprit. (See also *Mental Illness*)

Involuntary Mental Hospitalization

The criminal in prison loses his liberty, but not his credibility. While in prison, Bertrand Russell wrote a well-received book, and Nelson Mandela prepared himself to become the leader of his country.

The mental patient in a psychiatric facility loses both his liberty and his credibility. In effect, he is sentenced to a life-long loss of his "voice": regardless of what he says, people no longer "hear" it as the uttering of a full-fledged human being; instead they "interpret" it as the "symptom" of a lunatic's "brain disease." (See also *Mental Hospitalization*)

Irrational, Irrationality

Philosophers, psychiatrists, and lay persons alike regularly use the term "irrational" without defining its meaning.

A is likely to call B's belief and behavior irrational whenever A strongly disagrees with B's belief or rejects B's behavior as self-destructive or unwise. In short, when A calls B irrational, what he really means is: "I am rational and B is not like me."

What counts as rational belief and behavior compared with B's conduct, which is deemed to be irrational? It is the belief and behavior of A's group or profession or the society both A and B inhabit.

Atheists are likely to label religious beliefs and rituals "irrational."

Educated people are likely to label beliefs based on ignorance or superstition—for example, the belief that the earth is flat or the number 13 is unlucky—"irrational."

Psychiatrists are likely to label certain patterns of behavior they and society condemn—for example, anti-Semitism, racism, criminality—"irrational."[7] (See also *Mental Illness*, *Rationality*)

Isms

Communism, Nazism, Zionism, Islamism, Nationalism—all isms are the sworn enemies of clear thinking, tolerance, and liberty.

J

Jews

John Gross, long-time editor of the *Times Literary Supplement*: "To be Jewish is to belong to a club from which there is no resigning."[1]

Jewishness is a congenital stigma. Schizophrenia is an acquired stigma. Both are ineradicable.

* * *

In the educated, upward-mobile social milieu of Budapest in which I grew up, the great majority of Jews regarded being Jewish as a stigmatizing birthmark, an unsightly blemish they did not choose and had no reason to preserve.

Those who thought the stigma could be successfully removed by cosmetic conversion to Catholicism, converted. Those who didn't, remained "Jewish" agnostics and atheists. Those who thought it was not a stigma, embraced the identity.

Joy

The greatest joy is loving one's daughter or son. The second greatest is being loved in return.

K

Killing

We are steadily replacing the idea that persons kill with the idea that mental illnesses kill.

We attribute both suicide and murder to mental illnesses, psychiatric drugs, and psychiatrists who fail properly to treat dangerous mental patients.

Knowledge/Ignorance

People in Germany did not know and still do not know that during the Nazi period, psychiatrists were exterminating mental patients by starvation, fatal injection, and gassing.

People in France did not know and still do not know that during the Nazi period, psychiatrists were exterminating mental patients by starvation.

Norbert Wiener—child prodigy, father of cybernetics, one of the genuine geniuses of the modern age—did not know he was Jewish until he went to college. He wrote:

> You may ask how it was possible for an intelligent boy like me to have any doubts about this when my grandmother Wiener as far back as I could remember had received a newspaper printed in what I knew to be Hebrew characters.... Furthermore, my cousin Olga had once told me that we were Jews; but my mother had contradicted this at a time when I had not yet learned to question the word of my parents.[1]

The most powerful incentive for knowledge is wanting to know; for ignorance, not wanting to know.

L

Language

In the animal kingdom, the rule is, eat or be eaten; in the human kingdom, define or be defined.

* * *

The struggle for definition is the struggle for life itself. In the typical western film, two men fight desperately for the possession of a gun that has been thrown to the ground. Whoever reaches the weapon first shoots and lives; his adversary is shot and dies.

In life, the struggle is for words, not guns: whoever first defines the situation is the victor; his adversary, the victim. For example, husband and wife, mother and child, do not get along. Who defines whom as mentally ill?

He who defines dominates and lives. He who is defined is subjugated and destroyed.

* * *

Naming is taming.

* * *

Choice is good; discrimination is bad.

* * *

Aphorism is to description as caricature is to portrait.

* * *

The microscope and the telescope are optical instruments constructed by means of the proper arrangement of lenses. An analogy is a conceptual instrument constructed by means of the proper arrangement of words.

If an object is too small or too far to be perceptible to the naked eye, we might be able to see it by viewing it through an optical instrument. Similarly, if an idea is emotionally too close or too far for us to perceive, we might be able to see it by viewing it through an analogy.

* * *

The language of the natural sciences, mathematics, is a useful tool: it enables us to see what is otherwise invisible. The language of the social sciences, literalized metaphors, is an impediment: it prevents us from seeing the obvious.

This is why in the natural sciences knowledge can be gained only with the mastery of their special languages, whereas in human affairs, knowledge can be gained only by rejecting the pretentious jargons of the social sciences.

* * *

Metaphor is a verbal cartoon. We must grasp it, not analyze it.

* * *

"The greatest thing by far," says Aristotle, "is to be a master of metaphor. It is the one thing that cannot be learnt from others."[1]

Nowhere is the human fear of freedom displayed more tragically than in the one-sided application of this profound truth. Persons who create vivid metaphors and use them literally to enslave others—for example, Marx and Freud—are acclaimed as liberators, whereas those who unmask and mock the literalized metaphors of oppressors and liberate others—for example, Karl Kraus and Henry Mencken—are belittled as ignoble cynics.

* * *

Lord Palmerston cautioned: "Half the wrong conclusions at which mankind arrive are reached by the abuse of metaphors."[2]

But how do we know, who decides, whether a metaphor is used or abused? Is it used or abused in the Bible? In the story of the origin of the Ten Commandments? In the doctrine of transubstantiation? In the libido theory?

Time and again, we come back to the realization that if controlling man is the destination, the road to it lies through the control of language.

* * *

Bracketed as art, metaphor is poetry; bracketed as witticism, humor; bracketed as worship, religion; and bracketed as insanity, illness.

* * *

The immigrant who wants to live in a new language, not just speak it, must let a part of himself die. The self generated by the new language is a radically new self.

Refusal to learn the majority language is existential self-preservation or self-mutilation, depending on the immigrant's point of view.

* * *

We call coercing a woman to submit to a sexual act "rape."

We call coercing a person to submit to psychiatric defamation and confinement "diagnosis" and "treatment."

* * *

We call persons who harm children "child abusers."

We call persons who do not harm but value drugs, "drug abusers."

The term *drug abuse* is a linguistic symptom of the drug war's true agenda: persecuting the makers, sellers, and users of scapegoated drugs.

* * *

We call teenagers who have sex "sexually active."

We do not call teenagers who use drugs "pharmaceutically active." We call them "drug abusers."

* * *

Formerly, the young woman who engaged in sexual acts was called "promiscuous." Now, she is called "sexually active."

It is virtually impossible to describe human behavior without expressing approval or disapproval, praise or blame.

* * *

We call Americans who make money by selling drugs produced by chemists "drug company executives."

We call foreigners who make money by selling drugs produced by peasants "drug lords."

* * *

We call men who sell prescription drugs in drug stores "pharmacists."

We call men who sell illegal drugs on the street "pushers" and "criminals."

* * *

Jones gets divorced; we don't say he has lost his wife.

Jones kills himself; we say he has lost his life.

* * *

We don't call getting a speeding ticket "receiving police services"; getting audited by the Internal Revenue Service "receiving tax services"; or being indicted for a crime "receiving legal services."

But we call being involuntarily diagnosed as mentally ill and incarcerated in a mental hospital "receiving mental health services."

Accepting this usage precludes honest examination of the moral legitimacy of the psychiatric enterprise and dispassionate appraisal of the benefits and detriments of psychiatric coercions and excuses.

* * *

More than fifty years ago, C. S. Lewis lamented the increasing tendency to treat "mankind as mere specimens, preparations" and its effect on our language:

> Once we killed bad men: now we liquidate unsocial elements.... Most wonderful of all, the virtues of thrift and temperance, and even ordinary intelligence, are *sales-resistance*.[3]

Lewis did not live to see the day when the right to reject psychiatric assault is defined as "treatment resistance," and when "treatment resistance" and its management by forcibly drugging the "patient" form the subject of a new area of psychiatric expertise.

* * *

Quod licet Jovi, non licet bovi (What is permitted to Jove, is not permitted to the ox):

- Policemen receive bribes; politicians, campaign contributions.
- General Motors advertises automobiles; the American Psychiatric Association educates about mental illness.
- Marijuana is sold by pushers; tobacco, by merchants.
- The patient who goes to court to get out of the mental hospital is paranoid; the psychiatrist who goes to court to get him into the mental hospital is therapeutic.
- The patient who fakes illness malingers; the physician who fakes treatment practices psychotherapy or prescribes a placebo.
- Ingesting a prohibited drug is drug abuse; ingesting a prescribed drug is chemotherapy.
- The mental patient's explanation of his experience is a delusion; the psychiatrist's explanation of it is a diagnosis.

* * *

Medical mendacities masquerading as euphemisms:

- When one person forces another to work, we call it "slavery." When one person forces another to change his religion, we call it "forcible religious conversion." When one person forces another to submit to a sexual act, we call it "rape." When one person forces another to be incarcerated in a psychiatric institution, we call it "hospitalization," and when he forces another to ingest a psychiatric drug, we call it "treatment."
- Euthanasia: Physicians killing patients.
- Mental hospitalization: Psychiatrists imprisoning patients.
- Physician-assisted suicide: Physicians giving patients permission and a prescription to kill themselves.

- Planned parenthood: The prevention of parenthood.

* * *

Words as pretexts:

- Delusion: Pretext for incarcerating troublesome persons, calling it "mental hospitalization," and claiming it serves "the patients' best interests."

- Anti-psychotic medication: Pretext for evicting persons from mental hospitals, calling it "deinstitutionalization," and claiming it serves "the patients' best interests."

- Insanity defense: Pretext for depriving persons of responsibility and liberty, calling it "non-responsibility due to mental illness," and claiming it serves "the patients' best interests."

* * *

In inpatient (hospital) psychiatry, the best way to tell the patient from the psychiatrist is by who has the keys.

In outpatient (office) psychiatry, the best way to tell the patient from the psychiatrist is by who has the key words.

* * *

Ideologue: A person who uses ideas as incantations.

True believer: A person who accepts incantations as ideas.

Skeptic: A person who assumes that ideas are incantations until proven otherwise.

* * *

There are two kinds of screwdrivers, one for turning screws, another for drinking.

There are two kinds of patients, one for treating medically, another for coercing psychiatrically.

* * *

Language separates men from other animals. It also reduces persons to the level of animals, as in calling Jews "vermin" and policemen "pigs."

* * *

A person who feels sad may be said to be dejected or depressed. A person who claims to be God may be said to be boasting or deluded. The difference between these descriptions is the same as the difference between calling a spade a shovel or an agricultural implement for soil penetration, or between calling a man a "black" or a "nigger."

* * *

Language may be the original social contract. It seems likely that aboriginal man first vocalized idiosyncratically, each man making noise rather than speaking a language. When two or more individuals adapted their noisemaking to a common pattern, language was born.

All enduring customs may be based on the same mechanism.

* * *

Mathematics is a language lacking metaphors. That is why it is the perfect tool for conveying precise meaning (science), and why it is a perfectly useless tool for inspiring people (propaganda, poetry).

Music is a language of pure metaphor. That is why it is the perfect tool for moving people (religious or martial music), and why it is a perfectly useless tool for conveying any precise meaning whatever (speech).

* * *

The languages of religion and the so-called helping professions are comprised largely of literalized metaphors. That is why they are the perfect tools for legitimizing and illegitimizing ideas, behaviors, and persons.

* * *

Ordinary language combines the elements of all other "languages." It can be used literally and precisely, to convey meaning; metaphorically or poetically, to move people; or religiously, to blind and numb people, making them feel elevated or debased.

* * *

The war metaphor suggests a collective struggle against an adversary that deliberately attacks and seeks to destroy his opponent, typically a group or nation.

America wages war on drugs, crime, poverty, obesity, and mental illness. None of these things attack us, nor can we wage war against them.

The war against drugs and other metaphorical enemies conceals the real threat: personal responsibility. The war legitimizes the collective preference for state control over personal control of self-regarding behavior.

* * *

The American government could not prosecute the war on drugs without the active cooperation of the media, which systematically misdescribes crimes *due to the prohibition of drugs as due to the use of drugs.*

Crimes that violate drug prohibitions are systematically misdescribed as "drug-related." Al Capone's crimes were never characterized as "alcohol-related."

* * *

Racism: acknowledging the genetic differences among races; offensive speech, when spoken by whites about blacks, but not vice versa.

Sexism: acknowledging the genetic differences between the sexes; offensive speech, when spoken by men about women, but not vice versa.

* * *

Can a devout Catholic suffer from "clinical depression"? William F. Buckley, Jr. states: "Despair to a Catholic is itself a spiritual sin and blasphemy."[4]

* * *

A person asks me to explain why I believe that mental illness is a metaphor. I tell him. When he protests, "But that's *only* semantics," then I know I am not answering his question because he hasn't asked me a question.

* * *

Students of language have aptly noted that the ordinary man does not know that he speaks in prose.

Mutatis mutandis, the ordinary mental patient does not know that he speaks in metaphor.

The psychiatrist and the layman insist that he speaks in prose and conclude that the patient's assertions are the symptoms of mental illness.

* * *

The Greeks distinguished between language that enhanced and language that diminished persons, between noble and base rhetoric.

We fail to recognize that the terms we use to identify psychiatric illnesses and interventions are simply dysphemisms: base rhetoric to diminish persons.

* * *

Language, the oldest and still most reliable guide to a people's true sentiments, starkly reveals the intimate connections among illness, indignity, and illegitimacy.

In English, we use the same word to describe an expired passport, an indefensible argument, an illegitimate legal document, and a person disabled by disease: invalid.

To be an invalid, then, is to be an invalidated person, a human stamped "Not Valid" by the invisible but invincible hand of popular opinion. While invalidism carries with it the heaviest burden of indignity and illegitimacy, some stigma adheres to virtually all illness, to virtually any participation in the role of patient.

* * *

Peaceful atheists are often called "anti-religious."

Religious fanatics are never called "anti-atheists."

Ordinary language is incapable of being neutral toward important human affairs.

* * *

We love the addiction metaphor as a term of abuse.

We call people workaholics, chocaholics, foodaholics, shopaholics, drug addicts, exercise addicts, and sex addicts.

We never call people godaholics or religion addicts. We call them pious, fundamentalists, fanatics, zealots, and terrorists.

* * *

Persons who define others are like pathogenic microorganisms: they invade, parasitize, and often destroy their victims.

Individuals with poor social defenses—the young and the old, the sick and the poor—are most susceptible to being infected with invidious definitions of their identities.

* * *

"He who excuses himself, accuses himself," says a French proverb. The person who speaks in the language of excuses—blaming his misbehavior on addiction, disability, illness, mental illness, ignorance, poverty—begins the struggle for self-control by self-defeat.

* * *

The rhetoricians of drugs are not content with rejecting false claims about the harmfulness of certain drugs; they assert that toxic chemicals "expand the mind."

The rhetoricians of madness are not content with opposing psychiatric fraud and force; they maintain that madness "need not always be a breakdown, it can also be a breakthrough."[5]

Ours is the age in which partial truths are tirelessly transformed into total falsehoods and then acclaimed as revolutionary revelations.

* * *

"Words that are saturated with lies or atrocity," writes George Steiner, "do not easily resume life."[6]

This is what makes the languages of both madness and mad-doctoring rhetorics of deception and self-deception. The madman uses the rhetoric of "symptom"; the mad-doctor, the rhetoric of "diagnosis."

* * *

In 1961, at a hearing of a U.S. Senate Committee, Winfred Overholser, M.D., superintendent of St. Elizabeths Hospital in Washington, D.C., was asked: "[I]f I were eccentric...and I went to St. Elizabeths after having been thrown out of my boardinghouse...and said, 'I would like to be committed and have you look me over,' would you do it?"

Overholser: "We would not want to be used as a boardinghouse.... *We want some symptoms.*"[7]

The poor receive room and board in a mental hospital in exchange for symptoms, much as the rich receive room and board in a hotel in exchange for money.

* * *

For the Jew, God is Lord, not lord. A Lord cannot have a son, only a lord can. The Jewish God is pure metaphor.

For the Christian, God is both Lord and lord. He can have a son who is both man and God, lord and Lord. The Christian God is both metaphor and literalized metaphor.

* * *

"Homosexuality" is the name we give to the preference for sexual intercourse with members of one's own sex. For a long time, it was considered a serious mental illness.

Suppose we were to call preference for marriage with members of one's own race and religion "homoraciality" and "homoreligiosity." Would that make them mental illnesses? Should members of the American Psychiatric Association vote on whether or not they are mental illnesses?

* * *

Had the white settlers in North America called the natives "Americans" instead of "Indians," they could not have said that "the only good Indian is a dead Indian," and could not have deprived them so easily of their lands and lives.

Robbing people of their proper names is often the first step to robbing them of their property, liberty, and life.

* * *

When the Swiss are for nonintervention in war, they are called "neutral."

When Americans are for nonintervention, they are called "isolationists."

* * *

Our body is composed of what we eat; our mind, of what we hear, read, say, and write.

Insofar as others control what we can and cannot ingest, they control our body.

Insofar as others control what we can and cannot hear, read, say, and write, they control our mind.

Every society seeks to control what its members can and cannot take into their bodies and minds. The more such controls society exercises, the less free are its members.

* * *

As organisms or bodies, we live in physical space; as persons or minds, in linguistic space.

This is why a country is a matter of geography, but a nation a matter of language.

* * *

All higher organisms are territorial. That is, to survive, animals need physical territory or turf, and they struggle for it. We too are animals, and struggle for our turf, which has both physical and non-physical (spiritual) aspects.

To survive as spiritual beings or persons, we need a legitimate and secure spiritual-linguistic turf—a need manifested by our unceasing effort to make others share our religious fictions and adopt our linguistic conventions, worship our god, speak our language, and thus be "like-minded" persons.

* * *

We *use* things, but we *relate* to persons. Because we do not and should not use persons, we cannot properly speak of abusing them. Instead, we ought to speak of relating to them lovingly or hatefully, honestly or dishonestly, forgivingly or revengefully.

Phrases such as "child abuse," "wife abuse," "elder abuse"—modeled linguistically after terms such as "alcohol abuse"—reveal how deeply disrespectful we are toward the personhood of children and other powerless persons whose best interests we allegedly seek to protect.

* * *

Infants, idiots, the insane, and the ill *need* things. Healthy adults *want* things.

We speak in the language of needs when we address dependents, in the language of wants, when we address independent persons.

* * *

Verbal intercourse can be a form of existential intimacy more intense than sexual intercourse.

Conversation is more indispensable for personal survival than copulation.

* * *

Medicalized psychiatry denies the quintessential intimacy of verbal intercourse. Hence the obtuse conception of psychotherapy as something a doctor *gives* or *does* to a patient, as if it were like a surgical operation.

In surgery, all things being equal, doctor and patient are fungible. In psychotherapy, as in marriage or friendship, each person is a unique, irreplaceable individual.

* * *

Religions that cultivate other-worldliness, such as Christianity, extol the virtues of both celibacy and silence. Religions that do not, such as Judaism, extol the virtues of marriage and discourse.

The English word "parlor"—from the French *parler*, "to talk"—referred originally to a room in a monastery or nunnery where conversations were permitted, in particular between members of the religious order and visitors from the outside world.

* * *

We are rewarded or punished not for what we do, but for how our actions are interpreted by others. That is why often we are more interested in better justifying ourselves than in better behaving ourselves.

* * *

To concepts like suicide, homicide, and genocide, we should add "semanticide"—the murder of language. The deliberate or careless misuse of language, through hidden metaphor and professional mystification, breaks the basic contract between people: the tacit agreement on the proper use of words.

Celebrated philosophers and politicians whose aim was to control man—from Rousseau to Stalin—preached and practiced semanticide. As against them, celebrated writers—from Swift to Orwell—preached and practiced respect for language.

* * *

Mystification, exemplified by religion, moves multitudes.

Demystification, exemplified by science, influences individuals.

Law

Tacitus: "The more corrupt the state, the more laws it has."

* * *

The state cannot legalize an act; it can only prohibit it or leave it alone.

* * *

An old proverb cautions the would-be lawmaker not to prohibit what he cannot enforce. Modern American lawmakers follow the opposite rule: they are most zealous to prohibit that which they cannot enforce, exemplified by alcohol and drug prohibition.

* * *

If the person who breaks the law is not punished, the person who obeys it is cheated.

This is why lawbreakers ought to be punished: to encourage law-abiding behavior as useful and virtuous.

The aim of the criminal law cannot and must not be correction; it can only be, and ought to be, the maintenance of the legal order.

* * *

Today, punishment is unfashionable. Why? Because it creates moral distinctions among men, which, to the democratic mind, are odious.

We prefer a meaningless collective guilt to a meaningful individual responsibility.

* * *

There can be no humane penology so long as punishment masquerades as correction or treatment.

No person or group has the right to correct another adult. But persons and groups have the right to protect themselves by means of punishments, which may be as mild as a scolding or a small fine, or as harsh as life imprisonment or death.

* * *

A court of law has only one legitimate function: to justify coercion. It cannot be an organ of benevolence or "social justice."

Court-ordered remedies for social ills, such as mandating treatment for drug addicts or involuntarily hospitalized mental patients can only aggravate the problems they ostensibly seek to ameliorate.

* * *

I contend that psychiatric incarceration is always and necessarily a violation of human rights. Why? Because the psychiatric jailer, unlike the penological jailer, claims to be, and often sincerely believes himself to be, a legitimate double agent—protecting the patient from himself or from mental illness, and society from the patient.

Insofar as the psychiatrist is accepted as serving the patient's interests, the patient is deprived of legitimizing his grievance against the psychiatrist's treatment.

Insofar as the psychiatrist is accepted as serving society's interests, the psychiatrist is protected from legitimate criticism for depriving the patient of his liberty.

* * *

The very phrase, the "civil rights of mental patients," is an injury to their civil rights: it legitimizes the legal distinction between insane patients and sane citizens, *ipso facto* depriving the former of liberties and dignities enjoyed by the latter.

* * *

The civil rights of persons accused of mental illness will be protected only when people demand that civil rights be independent of psychiatric criteria, just as they are now independent of religious criteria; and when legislators and jurists deprive psychiatrists of the power to exercise social controls by means of seemingly medical interventions.

* * *

Laws regulating the use of potentially dangerous artifacts—such as automobiles, chainsaws, or drugs—ought to support, not supplant, self-controls.

Drug laws do exactly the opposite: they treat competent adults as undisciplined children rather than as responsible moral agents.

Legitimacy

Authority legitimizes; the individual justifies.

Legitimacy rationalizes; rationality legitimizes.

* * *

Legitimacy is weakened by defiance: that is why it seeks consensus and compliance, by persuasion, if possible, by coercion, if necessary.

Rationality is strengthened by defiance: that is why it is indifferent to consensus and eschews coercion.

* * *

Sources of legitimacy:

- God (Religion, the Church, the Pope)
- The Sovereign (Emperor, King, Monarch)
- The State (Parliament, the Law, the People)
- Tradition (Custom, "When in Rome do as the Romans do")
- Paternalism (Family, Parent, Expert)

- Dependency (Need, Illness, Poverty)
- Reason (Science, Medicine, Health)
- The Self (Individual rights, Autonomy)

* * *

What legitimizes one person's getting what he wants from another?

1. In the family: need. Responsible parents care for their children.
2. In Christianity and the welfare state: poverty. The poor are supported by the church or the state.
3. In totalitarian states and war: power. Rulers and victors extract what they want from the people and the vanquished.
4. In capitalism: money. Buyers purchase goods and services from sellers.

* * *

Legitimizing coercion:

- Affirmative action: Coercion in the name of justice.
- Involuntary psychiatric intervention: Coercion in the name of treatment.

* * *

The pen is said to be mightier than the sword. The sword needs the pen to legitimize it. We need the pen to distinguish between the *rightful* defense of God, country, and self and the *wrongful* killing of innocent people.

* * *

Physicians believe that there are two types of pains: physical and mental. Physical pain is caused by a bodily lesion, mental pain is caused by the mind.

Physicians do not experience other people's feelings; hence, properly speaking, they cannot classify their *pains.*

What they can and do classify are other people's *complaints.* Complaints of pain that physicians consider legitimate, they validate as "physical," those they consider illegitimate, they invalidate as "mental."

It is an error to believe that "organic pain" is one kind of pain, and "psychogenic pain" is another, the former standing in the same relation to the latter as, say, ureteral colic stands to biliary colic.

Instead, organic pain is a medically legitimate complaint, psychogenic pain, a medically illegitimate complaint, the former standing in the same relation to the latter as, say, legal tender stands to counterfeit.

Bodily pain is redeemable for a prescription for an opiate, mental pain is not.

* * *

Psychiatrists legitimize and delegitimize claims by examining the mind of the person who makes the assertion, not the evidence for the claim.

* * *

Because we are spiritual-social beings, our need for legitimacy is just as important as our need for food, water, and life itself. Sometimes it is even more important.

There are times when a person wants to die. There is never a time when a person wants to be illegitimate.

Illegitimacy is an ascription no one attributes to himself. Even the person guilty of a grave moral sin or crime—Judas, Lady Macbeth, Hitler, Stalin—does not view himself as an *illegitimate person.*

Legitimacy is the milieu in which we, as spiritual beings, live. To us it is what water is to fish: we notice it only when we are deprived of it (typically, by being incarcerated in a mental hospital).

* * *

Because man is a social animal, he must live in a group and secure a measure of cohesion in it. The easiest way to do so is by means of dramatic persecution of the Other—in Crusades, witch hunts, wars on enemies and drugs and mental illness.

Because man is a moral agent with a sense of right and wrong, he must legitimize his existential cannibalism. The easiest way to do so is by means of the dual claim that the control/destruction of the Other is necessary (1) to protect the purity and safety of the group, and (2) to save the soul/mental health of the Other.

How are these rationalizations supported? In the Age of Faith, by appeals to God, belief in immortality, and prayer for the Other's soul. In the Age of Reason, by appeals to medicine, belief in mental health, and the expenditure of vast sums on "treating" the Other's mind.

* * *

Why do we want to know whether or not depression is a scientifically proven disease, whether psychotherapy or psychoanalysis is a scientifically "valid" treatment? In part, because we need to decide whether insurance companies should or should not pay for such a service.

Confusing legitimacy with science and marrying medicine to the state corrupt both medicine and science.

* * *

In the nineteenth century, people saw the differences between legitimacy and rationality more clearly than they do today.

With the odor of sanctity lingering in their nostrils, people remembered and recognized that legitimacy allied with power is coercive, while rationality allied with knowledge is not.

Having replaced God with science, modern man believes that rationality legitimizes power and regards as legitimate the coercive control of persons and states deemed "irrational."

* * *

Asked by his secretary what he would have done had he lived in Spain under the Inquisition, Voltaire replied: "I would have worn a big rosary, and gone to mass every day and kissed all monks' sleeves, and tried to set fire to all their monasteries."[8] *Voila l'homme!*

Voltaire understood that only he who is legitimate can successfully wage war against the legitimizers.

Libertarians

"Political freedom means the absence of coercion of a man by his fellow man. The fundamental threat to freedom is power to coerce, be it in the hands of a monarch, a dictator, an oligarchy, or a momentary majority."[9]

In the everyday life of an ordinary American, the person most likely to possess power and use coercion against him is a psychiatrist. Yet, neither libertarians nor other writers on liberty acknowledge this.

In Victorian England, homosexuality was "the love that does not dare to speak its name." In the United States today, the liberty that does not dare to speak its name is the freedom to reject psychiatry.

If libertarians really meant that political freedom means the absence of coercion of a man by his fellow man, they would be more interested in psychiatry, where everything remains to be done, than in free-market economics, where the work is finished.

Liberty

Liberty and equality are at perpetual war with each other. Liberty fosters inequality. Inequality demands curtailing liberty in the name of equality. Loss of liberty fosters demands for freedom.

* * *

Liberty is having the right to believe in the divinity of Jesus as well as in the divinity of one's self; that is, having the right to be pious or psychotic. Beliefs injure no one. Only behaviors do that.

* * *

Liberty is what many people want for themselves and few want for others.

* * *

People love liberty because it protects them from control and humiliation by others, affording them the possibility of dignity.

People loathe liberty because it throws them back on their own abilities and resources, thus confronting them with the possibility of insignificance and the burden of responsibility.

* * *

If you truly yearn to be free, you must first recognize all the ways you are unfree. Only after constructing a complete catalogue of the constraints upon you can you begin to consider which ones you can and want to diminish or eliminate and at what cost (to you and others you cherish).

Your self-liberation will be complete when you are left with constraints to which you willingly, perhaps even eagerly, submit.

Library

Libraries: The scholars' laboratories.

* * *

Libraries: Oases in the desert of life.

Lies

Man lives in a sea of lies. Truth, like air to fish, is a toxin to him.

A few persons train themselves to tolerate small quantities of truth, under carefully controlled conditions, called atheism, science, skepticism.

Socrates said the unexamined life is not worth living and prescribed mind-expanding dialogues to help man get to know himself.[10]

Today, many people feel they cannot afford the luxury of examining their lives and psychiatrists prescribe mind-numbing chemicals to help them hide from themselves.

* * *

People who habitually lie to others also lie to themselves, eventually with disastrous consequences.

* * *

A Hungarian proverb warns: "Tell the truth and get your head bashed in."

Only in free and egalitarian situations can a person speak truthfully.

* * *

The psychiatrist interprets the patient's lies as delusions. Abolishing the lie, he abolishes language, and, abolishing language, he abolishes man, as C. S. Lewis warned that he would.[11]

* * *

Disraeli said: "There are three kinds of lies: lies, damned lies, and statistics."

In the therapeutic state, there are also three kinds of lies: lies, damned lies, and "clincal studies."

Editorial, *Journal of the American Medical Association*, 1948: "Extensive scientific studies have proved that smoking in moderation...does not appreciably shorten life. Postmortem examinations do not reveal lesions in any number of cases that could be definitely traced to the smoking of cigarettes...there does not seem to be any preponderance of evidence that would indicate the abolition of the use of tobacco as a substance contrary to the public health."[12]

Life

Life is a big empty hole. One of the best ways to fill it is by striving for and achieving excellence in the pursuit of one's chosen vocation.

* * *

Life is a bad joke God plays on us. Some take the joke too seriously—they are the madmen; others don't take it seriously enough—they are the humorists.

Most people think life is not a joke: they are the normal persons.

* * *

Persons whose lives are insignificant look for significance in the past or the future. Some find it in a mythologized religious, racial, or national past; others, in a utopian future for their children, nation, or mankind.

* * *

"The problem," says Gabriel Josipovici, "is to walk in God's way when that way is so badly mapped out."[13] If so, it is inconceivable that a stranger—let alone a group of strangers called an "institution"—could be our guide.

We must find the Way in our own souls, by cultivating autonomy and responsibility.

* * *

Happiness: tranquil illusion that life is worth living.
Sadness: tranquil recognition that life is not worth living.
Mania: frenzied version of happiness.
Depression: frenzied version of sadness.

* * *

Most people cannot accept that life is a continuous burden and the need to cope with it never ends.

Litigation

The frequency and outcome of personal injury litigation in the United States are best viewed as manifestations of a translation, into the American language of capitalism, of Marx's famous maxim, "From each according to his ability, to each according to his need."

* * *

Smokers sue tobacco manufacturers—for not warning them that smoking increases their chances of developing lung cancer.

Adolescents sue the manufacturers of fast foods—for not warning them that gluttonous consumption of their product increases their chances of becoming obese.

Pregnant adolescents ought to sue God, the manufacturer of their genital apparatus—for not warning them that its use without contraception increases their chances of becoming pregnant.

The logic of American product liability litigation: *Caveat vendor.*

Location

The maxim for the successful retailing of goods is: "Location, location, location." The same is true for the retailing of ideas. One requires favorable physical space, the other, favorable cultural space. Each location must abound with individuals interested in and able to afford what the seller is marketing.

Logic

Proving what's false is easy; proving what's obvious, impossible.

Loneliness

People don't fear being dead, they fear being alone. That is why hell is full of people, demons, and tumult. Being the victim of eternal torment signifies that someone cares enough about you to torment you. *Ergo*, you are not alone, you are not unimportant, you exist.

The fear of being alone is emblematic of our social nature. Descartes said: *Cogito, ergo sum* ("I think, therefore I am"). It would be more accurate to say: "*You exist, therefore I am.*"

* * *

"Hell," declared Sartre, "is other people." But he abhorred being alone.

* * *

The lonely person is like an actor onstage, eager to display his talents, staring down into the abyss of a dark and empty theater.

When he fills the emptiness with an imaginary crowd of theatergoers eager to see him perform, he is declared to be a lunatic.

Looking

Pleasure from looking at:

- nature: a naturalist
- paintings in a museum: a connoisseur or collector of art
- pornography: a pervert
- sex acts and organs: a voyeur
- stamps: a philatelist

Love

The child loves out of dependency; the lover, out of lust; the newlywed, out of duty; the spouse and the parent, out of devotion; the long married and the grandparent, out of habit.

* * *

We should love our children more than they love us, and even when they don't love us, because their sense of self and self-esteem depends on our love more than ours depends on their love.

But we should not love our spouses or lovers more than they love us, lest they misinterpret devotion as dependence.

* * *

In the past parents and children *loved* each other; now they *bond*.

* * *

Infants love the person who feeds them. Adults love the food that relieves their hunger or pleases their palate, not the person who cooks or serves it.

However, adults are expected to love their partners who satisfy their sexual hunger, not their sexual partner's erotic attributes.

* * *

Men and women "in love" share the mistaken belief that they live in the same world. They come to "love" one another when they acknowledge that they live in different worlds, but are prepared, once in a while, to cross the chasm that separates them.

M

Madness

"The madman," said Gilbert K. Chesterton, "is not the man who has lost his reason. The madman is the man who has lost everything except his reason."[1] He was right.

"The madman," we say, "is not himself; he has lost control over himself." We are wrong and arrogant: We authorize psychiatrists to tell him who he is, by giving him a diagnosis; and to control him, by incarcerating and drugging him, "in his own best interest."

* * *

Chesterton's remark is profoundly wise. *If you give up everything except your reason, then others—especially members of your family—are likely to call you "mad."* The Gospels present precisely this scenario about Jesus. Having withdrawn from society, Jesus goes about the land preaching and defying what the Jews view as the law of God:

> And he entered again into the synagogue: and there was a man there with a withered hand. And they watched him, whether he would heal him on the sabbath day: that they might accuse him.... For he had healed many: insomuch as they pressed upon him to touch him, as many as had plagues.... And when his friends heard of it, they went out to lay hold on him: for they said, "He is beside himself." (Mark 3: 1-2, 10, 21)

Brian Incigneri, a Catholic theologian in Australia, suggests this interpretation:

> The first appearance of Jesus' family in any of the Gospels occurs in Mark 3: 20-35, and it depicts them very negatively. They seem to be an obstacle to his mission. More than that, they seem to accuse him in the same way that the scribes do.... Mark 3: 21 may reflect a genuine memory of difficulties Jesus had with his family when, as a single Jewish man in his thirties, he left his family to go on the road to preach the Kingdom of God. Certainly, Mark

> 3: 20–35 paint a very unflattering picture of Jesus' family.... In v. 21 *his family accuses him of being "out of his mind."* Immediately following this, in v. 22, the scribes accuse him of being possessed by the devil. Both accusations are similar. In the ancient world, one who had a mental illness was commonly thought to be possessed by a devil. The accusation of his family is like the accusation of the scribes.[2]

By calling Jesus "mad," his family and the scribes try to discredit him and persuade people to not listen to him. This has always been and still is the essential prescriptive meaning of the term "mad" (and its modern variants).[3]

* * *

Bertrand Russell showed a keen sensitivity to the close connections between madness and power, but a remarkable insensitivity to the similar connections between psychiatry and power. He wrote:

> While animals are content with existence and reproduction, men desire also to expand, and their desires in this respect are limited only by what imagination suggests as possible. *Every man would like to be God, if it were possible; some few find it difficult to admit the impossibility. These are the men framed after the model of Milton's Satan, combining, like him, nobility with impiety. By "impiety" I mean something not dependent upon theological beliefs: I mean refusal to admit the limitations of individual human power....*
>
> The love of power is a part of normal human nature, but power-philosophies are, in a certain precise sense, insane. The existence of the external world, both that of matter and that of other human beings, is a datum, which may be humiliating to a certain kind of pride, but can only be denied by a madman. Men who allow their love of power to give them a distorted view of the world are to be found in every asylum: one man will think he is the Governor of the Bank of England, another will think he is the King, and yet another will think he is God. Highly similar delusions, if expressed by educated men in obscure language, lead to professorships of philosophy; and if expressed by emotional men in eloquent language, lead to dictatorships. *Certified* lunatics are shut up because of their proneness to violence when their pretensions are questioned; the *uncertified* variety are given the control of powerful armies, and can inflict death and disaster upon all sane men within their reach. The success of insanity, in literature, in philosophy, and in politics, is one of the peculiarities of our age, and the successful form of insanity proceeds almost entirely from impulses towards power."[4]

Yet, Russell persecuted his only son, John, with psychiatrists and had him incarcerated as a madman.[5]

* * *

Madness was not a problem or a puzzle for the ancients or for Shakespeare.

By fostering the false belief that relations among reasonable people are harmonious, the Enlightenment turned madness into a mystery.

Inharmonious relations, especially in the family, became perceived as madness qua "unreasonableness" on the part of certain "unreasonable" persons. At the same time, people learned to avoid using plain language in speaking about the (mis)behavior of "unreasonable" persons, and adopted instead the hushed tones and mystical vocabulary appropriate to discourse about an unfathomable mystery.

The more we claim to want to understand what *the mad person thinks about himself*, the better we succeed at not understanding what *we think about our reaction to him*, and the greater grows the mystery of his "madness." (See also *Mental Illness*)

Marriage

Romantic love rests largely on loneliness and lust. This is why it is so poor a basis for marriage, which must rest largely on affection and respect.

* * *

Women marry hoping their husbands will change; men, hoping their wives won't. This is bad enough. Couples can make it much worse by going to a psychiatrist to fix the problem.

* * *

Marriage is:

1. Existential "self-medication" to combat loneliness.
2. A side effect of the desire for coitus.
3. A gift a man gives to a woman for which she never forgives him.
4. Tenured togetherness.
5. The belated discovery of having made a huge mistake.

6. A human relationship that begins as an act of mutual sexual legitimation, called "making love," and often ends as an act of mutual existential deligitimation, called "divorce."

7. A legally binding contract the contracting parties are expected to enter (the first time) without legal assistance, but cannot exit without it.

* * *

Marriages are made in Heaven. That's why they don't work here on Earth.

* * *

Every marriage is an interpersonal "arrangement." We should distinguish not between marriages and arrangements, but among different types of marital and nonmarital arrangements.

* * *

Marriage is merging lives. Sex is merging bodies. Combining them is hazardous to happiness.

That is why religions sanctify marriage as blessed and holy, and condemn fornication as messy and unholy.

* * *

Successful marriage depends more on husband and wife wanting to merge their lives and fortunes than on their loving each other.

* * *

The institution of marriage was not made to last as long as married people now last.

* * *

Women are now on equal existential and legal footing with men. They no longer need, nor deserve, the sort of legal protection that traditional marriage provided them.

Sexual relations between consenting adults are now protected by law as a basic human right. Hence, the state no longer has the sort of political interest in monitoring marriage as it had in the past.

If this is so, state licensure of marriage is scarcely more justified than state licensure of sexual relations outside of marriage. Perhaps the time is near for the state to cease recognizing marriage as an institution, leaving that function to religion, and treat marriage as a private matter, similar to a private economic relationship.

* * *

A married couple is a whole that often is less than the sum of its parts.

* * *

A metaphor for many a modern marriage: Two competent swimmers in the water, safe but solitary, decide to play: One pretends to drown, the other to rescue; they grapple, sink, panic, and drown together.

* * *

By becoming "one body" in marriage, wives can injure their husbands by eating too much, and husbands can injure their wives by drinking too much.

What psychiatrists call "self-destructive behavior" may be exactly the opposite: an attempt to preserve one's identity by impairing or trying to rid oneself of one's "parasite."

* * *

Alimony: Restitution payment to compensate the victim for the ravages of matrimony.

* * *

In intimate human relations, personal autonomy and physical proximity tend to be incompatible.

Persons who want to maximize both, especially in marriage, are likely to have neither. Those who are satisfied with some of each—as married people used to be—sometimes may end up with one or the other or sometimes both.

* * *

When a marriage becomes intensely unsatisfactory, the participants have a choice between breaking up or breaking down. Some prefer the former, others, the latter. Either solution is likely to generate new problems.

Sometimes, the breakup of the marriage leads to the breakdown of the wife or the husband. Often, the breakdown of the wife or the husband leads to a "stronger" marriage, the sick member's partner assuming the role of the nurse-protector of his or her insane partner. The marriage between Leonard and Virginia Woolf is an example.

* * *

Traditional, arranged marriage was a fine institution for legitimizing men and women as adults and for raising children. It could be ruined, and often was ruined, by the expectation that the participants enjoy each other as sexual partners.

Modern, romantic marriage is a fine institution for legitimizing men and women as adults and for companionship and sex. It can be ruined, and often is ruined, by the expectation that the participants will have children whom they will love and protect.

* * *

There are two ways of terminating a marriage.

One is to draw up a set of grievances against one's partner, much as a grand jury draws up a set of criminal indictments against a defendant. The "accuser" can then use these "offenses" to justify detaching himself from his partner.

The other is to accept being mismatched with one's partner and gradually withdraw from the commitment. The relationship will then wither away.

Martyr

Webster's defines "martyr" as a person who suffers death as the penalty for "refusing to renounce a religion," or who sacrifices "life itself for the sake of principle," or, generally, a person condemned to great and chronic suffering, as in "a martyr to asthma all his life."

In modern usage, the term "martyr" implies persecution and injustice committed by the powerful, suffered by the powerless.

Heretics were martyrs to religious persecution; black victims of lynching were martyrs to racial persecution; persons imprisoned for possessing illegal drugs are martyrs to pharmacratic persecution. The only persecuted people not considered martyrs are mental patients incarcerated in insane asylums, subjected to destructive "treatments."

Anne Frank is a martyr. Rosemary Kennedy is not.[6]

Why? Because the "diagnosis" and "treatment" of "mental illness" is *never considered unjust*. If such interventions are condemned at all, they are criticized as *mistakes, not as injustices*.

* * *

The person who martyrs himself is more likely to do so because his attachment to people is weak, than because his faith in a cause is strong.

Media

In the theological state, the media becomes the voice of clerical orthodoxy and eagerly assumes the job of delegitimizing the voices of the critics of religious correctness.

In the therapeutic state, the media becomes the voice of clinical orthodoxy and eagerly assumes the job of delegitimizing the voices of the critics of medical, especially psychiatric, correctness.

Medicalization

People used to be mistaken about their health and disagreed with their doctors. Now they are "in denial."

Medical Ethics

The three justifications for medical intervention: pathology, permission, paternalism. In other words, treatment may be premised on illness, consent, or "benevolent" coercion.

* * *

There is enough infection and death in the world; under no circumstances should the physician himself infect and kill his patient. To Ignaz Semmelweis, that seemed like elementary obstetrical ethics.

Mutatis mutandis, there is enough coercion and unfreedom in the world; under no circumstances should the physician (psychiatrist) coerce and render his patient unfree. To me, this seems like elementary psychiatric ethics.

* * *

When a person claims to be sick while his physician considers him physically healthy, he is said to be "neurotic."

When a person claims to be well while his physician considers him mentally ill, he is said to be "psychotic" and "treatment-resistant."

In the medical ethic, the patient must have the physician's permission to assume the sick role as well as to reject it.

In the libertarian ethic, the patient is free to assume or reject the sick role as he wishes. It is not the physician's role to regulate the patient's behavior; his role is to regulate his own behavior, that is, decide whether to accept or not accept a person who seeks his help as *his* patient.

* * *

The ethics of pharmacracy does not destroy the concept of responsibility, it perverts it: it excuses personal failure by attributing it to bad genes, bad parents, or bad social conditions, but credits personal achievement by attributing it to creativity, hard work, and free will.

* * *

The death of virtue:

1. William Bennett encourages high school students "to tell on their friends.... 'It isn't snitching or betrayal to tell an adult that a friend of yours is using drugs and needs help. It's an act of true loyalty—of true friendship.'"[7]

2. Mental health professionals call wickedness "illness."

* * *

The death of love in the family: calling the relatives whose imprisonment they plot "loved ones." "Committing a loved one can be the best medicine.... Commitment can be an empowering process for people with mental illness."[8]

Medicine

Formerly, when religion was strong and science weak, men mistook magic for medicine; now, when science is strong and religion weak, men mistake medicine for magic.

* * *

Formerly, a quack was someone who had fake cures for real diseases; now, he is someone who claims to have real cures for fake diseases.

* * *

Formerly, people were duped by quacks because they believed in their fake cures; now, they are duped by them because they believe in their fake diseases.

* * *

Formerly, when our religion was Christianity, we fasted and feasted; now that our religion is medicine, we diet and binge.

Thus was gluttony replaced by obesity, prayer by psychotherapy, the monastery by the clinic, the clergyman by the clinician, the Vatican by the Food and Drug Administration, and God, for whom being slim meant being virtuous, by medicine, for which it means being healthy.

* * *

Formerly, when religion ruled the mind of man, people believed in word magic. Prayer possessed boundless power to save man; blasphemy, boundless power to damn him.

Today, when medicine rules the mind of man, people believe in drug magic. Drugs prescribed by doctors possess boundless powers to cure; drugs prohibited by doctors, boundless powers to sicken.

Our images of divine and devilish powers have remained the same; only the objects to which they are attributed have changed, from words in the theological state, to drugs in the therapeutic state.

* * *

How can a layperson now distinguish medicine from religion, medical treatment from faith healing?

He cannot tell by who benefits, nor by the methods used. The only way he can tell is by observing whether the state pays for it. If it does, it's medicine and treatment; if it doesn't, it's religion and faith healing.

* * *

If a person wants something, called a "lesion," removed from his body, he must go to a doctor and *give* him written permission for it; this is called giving "informed consent for surgery."

If a person wants something, called a "prescription drug," added to his body, he must go to a doctor and *obtain* his written permission for it; this is called getting a "prescription."

* * *

Third-party payment for medical services has transformed the practice of medicine from the *healing of persons* into the *production of health*.

This misapplication of assembly line techniques to the doctor-patient relationship creates dissatisfied doctors, unhappy patients, and deteriorating health care despite technical advances in medicine.

* * *

The greatest analgesic, soporific, stimulant, tranquilizer, narcotic, and even antibiotic known to medicine—in short, the closest thing to a genuine panacea—is work.

* * *

We call the Pope "pontiff," from the Latin *pontifex* or "bridge builder" (from *pons* and *facere*), to signify that he is our ultimate bridge from this world to the next.

Now, the physician is our pontiff, the bridge from a world of illness to one of health.

The clerical pontifex enabled the dead soul to ascend to heaven. The clinical pontifex enables the sick to ascend to health.

Thus do we re-theologize medicine.

* * *

Religion gives meaning to life; medicine does not. The modern tendency to theologize health is a futile attempt to cling simultaneously to the practices and promises of both religion and science. People who do that risk reaping the bitterest fruits of both harvests.

* * *

Justifications for treatment:

- For the true believer in medicine: disease.
- For the medical autocrat: the need for treatment.
- For the loyal pharmacrat: a court order.
- For the libertarian: the patient's consent.

Ignoring or confusing these conflicting moral premises is the source of most of our problems in medical ethics.

* * *

Symptom, sign, disease:

A symptom—for example, fatigue or pain—is said to be subjective. A sign—for example, fever or high blood pressure—is said to be objective. Although this is a fair approximation to what is at stake here, the subjective/objective dichotomy may mislead.

Both symptoms and signs are *reports* a person makes about a body. Typically, a symptom is a report the patient makes about his own body, whereas a sign is a report someone other than the patient makes about the patient's body. Both may be true or false.

A symptom may be false because the patient often has good reasons to deceive doctors and others. A sign may be false because physicians or laboratory technicians often make errors.

* * *

Frequently, patients with obscure complaints—for example, veterans with so-called Gulf War Syndrome—seek the help of the physician.

In many such cases, the physician cannot find any medical—that is, patho-anatomical or pathophysiological—causes for the complaints.

Today, medical etiquette and the need to conform to the profession's "standard of care" prevent the physician from saying to the patient: "Mr. Jones, I have examined you as best as I know how, and I have done all the tests, as indicated by your problem. I must frankly tell you, I do not know what is wrong with you. I am very sorry that I cannot be of further help to you."

Instead, the physician attributes the patient's problem to anxiety, depression, stress, or mental illness and refers him to a mental health professional.

* * *

Criteria for successful treatment:

If medical intervention is based on complaint, the result must be measured in terms of the patient's satisfaction with the intervention.

If medical intervention is based on lesion, the result must be measured in terms of lesion-removal and/or restoration of function.

Quacks do a better job removing complaints, surgeons at removing lesions.

* * *

Until recent times, a seriously ill person either recovered or died. Biotechnological advances have created three radically different outcomes of medical treatment and three correspondingly different aims for medical intervention:

1. Enabling the patient to live as a socially functioning, self-respecting person.

2. Transforming the sick person into a chronic, "professional" patient, dependent on doctors and others.

3. Keeping the patient alive as a quasi-cadaver, physicians demonstrating their ability to keep organs and tissues alive.

* * *

If you free a person of his obligation to pay for his treatment, you also deprive him of his right to define what constitutes treatment.

Collectivistic planners for health care services, acting in defiance of the proverbial rule that "he who pays the piper calls the tune," sow the wind of medical idealism, but reap the whirlwind of medical indifference and incompetence.

* * *

Today, everyone claims to be working for the patient's best interests. No wonder the patient is in deep trouble.

Meme

Meme is a term coined in 1976 by Richard Dawkins, Simonyi Professor for the Public Understanding of Science, University of Oxford, which he defined as "a new replicator, a unit of cultural transmission, or a unit of imitation."[9]

The idea of the "meme" has generated the new quackery of memetics, much as the old idea of mental illness generated the old quackery of psychiatry.

Memeticians, who write in the *Journal of Memetics: Evolutionary Models of Information Transmission*, view the meme as "a contagious information pattern that replicates by parasitically infecting human minds and altering their behavior, causing them to propagate the pattern. Individual slogans, catch-phrases, melodies, icons, inventions, and fashions are typical memes. An idea or information pattern is not a meme until it causes someone to replicate it, to repeat it to someone else."[10]

Creating new words can lead to ignorance as well as to knowledge.

Memory

Memory is the ability to remember what never happened, and forget what has happened.

Men

It took men thousands of years to discover that women are human.

It took women only a few decades to discover that men are not.

Mental Health Services

Psychiatrists pleading for more publicly-funded mental health services is a classic case of what economists call "rent seeking": a demand for more tax monies for mental health professionals, ostensibly to satisfy the growing need of their "beneficiaries," who in fact are their victims.

Mental Hospital

"People fear witches, and burn women," observed Justice Louis Brandeis.[11]

People fear the mentally ill, and deprive innocent persons of liberty.

* * *

The medical hospital is a repair shop.
The mental hospital is a parking place.

* * *

For the inmate who enters voluntarily or conspires in his own commitment: an existential parking place.

For the inmate "hospitalized" against his will by his "loved ones": a junk heap for the family's discarded relatives.

* * *

Involuntary mental hospitalization is psychiatric slavery.

Refining the legal or psychiatric criteria for commitment is like prettifying plantations.

The problem is not how to reform commitment laws, but how to abolish the practice of psychiatric coercion.

* * *

Mental hospitals are:

1. Orphanages for adult "orphans."

2. The POW camps of our undeclared and unarticulated family wars.

3. Parking places for people who want to get out of the traffic jams of life.

4. Cemeteries for the living dead: dormitory beds are the gravesites; psychiatric diagnoses, the gravestones; psychiatrists, the gravediggers; patients, the corpses. In the literal cemetery, microorganisms in the soil live off the tissues of the dead body; in the metaphorical cemetery, macroorganisms (mental health professionals) live off the spirit of the living patient.

* * *

As long as there are laws that authorize taxation, there can be no voluntary taxpayers. Similarly, as long as there are commitment laws, there can be no voluntary mental hospital patients.

Mental Illness

A glossary:

Ambivalence: Mixed feelings.

Compulsion: Persistent, self-administered command.

Delusion: Belief said to be false by persons who do not share it.

Elation: Self-exultation and self-glorification.

Insanity: Insubordination to civilian authority.

Multiple personality: The many false faces of the person unwilling to show his true face.

Narcissism: Conceit.

Obsession: Persistent self-administered idea, especially doubt or certainty.

Psychosis: Malignant seriousness manifested by inability to laugh at oneself.

* * *

Mental illness as drama:

Depression: Tragedy.

Hysteria: Melodrama.

Mania: Comedy.

Paranoia: Parody.

Transvestism: Farce.

* * *

Mental illness as caricature:

Depression: Contrition.

Grandiosity: Conceit.

Hypochondriasis: Concern for being healthy.

Mania: Decisiveness.

Obsession-compulsion: Conscientiousness.

Paranoia: Concern for danger and protection.

Schizophrenia: Indolence and lawlessness.

* * *

Mental illness as self-conversation:

Hypochondriasis: "I am sick. The doctors don't believe me. They can't find out what is wrong with me."

Depression: "I am worthless. I am no good to anyone. I might as well be dead."

Mania/bipolar illness: "I am a great person. Life is great. I am going to live it up."

Schizophrenia: "I am a talented and sensitive person, but no one appreciates me. I can't stay in school, the students and teachers are so crude and insensitive. I should stay home for a while and think."

Paranoia: "I have invented a cure for cancer but the drug companies refuse to buy my invention. Now the FBI is tapping my telephone."

Erotomania: "Robert Redford is in love with me. I know he is writing to me, but someone intercepts his letters."

* * *

Mental illness is the name of a category of alleged "conditions" that has no members.

There is no mental illness. There is a diversity of human behaviors, some socially approved, others socially disapproved. In modern societies, many people prefer to view some disapproved behaviors as diseases and call them "mental illnesses."

* * *

Mental illness is to psychiatry as phlogiston was to chemistry.

Establishing chemistry as a science of the nature of matter required the recognition of the nonexistence of phlogiston.

Establishing psychiatry as a science of the nature of human behavior requires the recognition of the nonexistence of mental illness.

* * *

Psychiatrists say that the homosexual who doesn't like being a homosexual suffers from an illness called "ego-dystonic homosexuality."

Psychiatrists do not say the Jew who doesn't like being Jewish suffers from an illness called "ego-dystonic Judaism"; or the woman who doesn't like being a woman, from an illness called "ego-dystonic femininity"; or the poor person who doesn't like being poor, from an illness called "ego-dystonic destitution."

* * *

Crime is illegal behavior. Mental illness is illegitimate behavior. By definition, illegal behavior is illegitimate.

It is not surprising that crime is increasingly viewed as mental illness, and that psychiatric sanctions increasingly replace criminal penalties.

* * *

Illness, mental illness, race, religion, occupation: each, *inter alia,* is a role that a person may assume willingly or that may be imposed on him against his will.

One of the features that distinguishes medical illness from mental illness—schizophrenia from anemia—is that mental illness defines the person, whereas medical illness does not.

This is why we read about "schizophrenic murderers," but not about "anemic murderers."

* * *

A woman kills her nine-month-old son because, she says, "The baby is the devil.... If I kill the demon, my husband will raise the baby to life again in three days and the world will know he is Jesus Christ."

Charged with first-degree murder, the woman is acquitted as not guilty by reason of insanity. She sues her obstetrician and the psychiatrist who had treated her during her pregnancy.[12]

Psychiatrists say she was suffering from postpartum psychosis. I say she is colossally conceited.

* * *

Mental illness is a problem for the patient's family and society. For the patient, it is a solution.

This was Freud's only discovery. Psychoanalysts ignore it, psychiatrists deny it.

* * *

The proverb counsels to light a candle, not curse the darkness. This advice overlooks the advantages of cursing the darkness and remaining in darkness, namely, the benefits of victimhood.

* * *

Today, the mental hospital patient has many rights, but no liberty. In the past, he had no rights, but more liberty: escape from the hospital, called "elopement," was easy.

* * *

Relationship with other human beings is a basic human need. Traditionally, this need has been met mainly by and within the family, stabilized by religion and tradition.

As family ties have loosened and persons have become true individuals, family relationships as sources of human contact have been replaced, in part, by what we call "chronic mental illness."

We are expected to see only the disutility of mental illness. Its utility lies in uniting family members no longer bound by parental, marital, or filial ties.

* * *

If a person does something dramatically bad—for example, shoots the president—we immediately assume that he might be mentally ill, as if mental illness were a reasonable explanation for his action.

If a person does something dramatically good—for example, saves a child from a burning building—we make no similar assumption.

No further evidence is needed to show that "mental illness" is not the name of a biological condition whose nature awaits to be elucidated, but the name of a concept whose purpose is to obscure the obvious.

* * *

We *discredit* the mad criminal as lacking criminal intent and do not blame him for his destructive crime, but we *credit* the mad artist with artistic intent and praise him for his artistic creation.

This disjunction is inconsistent with the idea that mental illness causes (criminal) behavior.

* * *

In 1988, an Arkansas appeals court ruled that "bipolar disorder is a physical, not mental, illness."

Commented Paul Fink, M.D., then president-elect of the American Psychiatric Association: "The Arkansas case gives psychiatrists an extraordinary window of opportunity."[13]

Psychiatrists look to judges, not pathologists, to validate that their diagnoses are diseases.

* * *

For more than two hundred years, until the middle of the twentieth century, psychiatrists and lay persons alike regarded satisfying one's need for sex by and for oneself—which they called "self-abuse" and we call "masturbation"—as the cause and consequence of serious mental illness. It took medical science and public opinion a long time to acknowledge that sexual self-satisfaction was a ubiquitous act, neither an illness nor the cause of one.

Today, psychiatrists and lay persons alike regard satisfying one's need for dialogue by and for oneself—which they call "hallucination" and "hearing voices," and I call "talking to oneself" or "verbal masturbation"—as the manifestation of serious mental illness that ought to be suppressed by whatever means necessary, including lobotomy, electric shock treatment, and antipsychotic drugs. Perhaps it will take even longer than it took for masturbation for medical science and public opinion to acknowledge that talking to oneself is a ubiquitous act, neither an illness nor the cause of one.

* * *

Manufacturing mental illness:

A Canadian politician's new disease: "Honorable senators, illiteracy touches probably more than 20 percent of our population.... It is not a partisan issue. It affects us all…[it] is truly a national disease…. [We] must understand that this is one disease that can be cured."[14] Spreading the alarm, a reporter in Ottawa adds: "Illiterates more commonly read the Bible and other religious material, while literates lean more to reference books, fiction, and manuals.[15]

* * *

A Florentine psychiatrist's new disease:

In a 182-page book titled "The Stendhal Syndrome," [Dr. Graziella] Magherini details the cases of 106 tourists admitted to Santa Maria Nuova Hospital in Florence in the last 10 years suffering from delirium, disorientation and paranoia brought on by exposure to magnificent works of art. Hundreds of milder cases, probably thousands more, have gone unreported.... "The worst case had to be in the hospital 10 days," said Magherini, head of the psychiatric ward at Santa Maria Nuova and a lecturer on psychiatry at the University of Florence.[16]

* * *

A psychiatry professor's new disease:

[T]he rush or the feeling that you get from this [combat addiction] is one of an addiction to adrenalin, addiction to cocaine…when I get into this high it is just like being in Vietnam, the thrill of killing, the thrill of destroying. And it's something I just cannot overcome, even with medication.... It's hard to duplicate this high with drugs, except the only drug I know is cocaine…[that gives you] the same type of high of killing, of destroying.[17]

* * *

A social worker's new disease:

> "I don't think there is any doubt Satanism is a growing problem," said social worker Dale Trahan, who has been researching Satanic beliefs for three years and was contracted to organize the program for the Treatment of Ritualistic Deviance.... Psychiatrists and psychologists at Hartgrove Hospital [in Chicago] are creating one of the nation's first treatment programs to wean teenagers away from Satanism.... [Teenagers] spend four to eight weeks as inpatients and undergo individual and group counseling.... The new program will seek to undermine Satanism's underlying belief system.[18]

* * *

Psychiatrists say that the woman who starves herself of food suffers from "anorexia nervosa."

Psychiatrists do not say the man who starves himself of sex suffers from "anerotica nervosa."

Why not? Because they are cowards and hypocrites: they fear the wrath of the Church that would view their diagnosis as a defamation of celibacy.

The Church defines celibacy as "a gift from God." If psychiatrists were to define it as anerotica nervosa it would be a mental illness requiring psychiatric treatment.

* * *

Mental diseases stand in the same relation to bodily diseases as enslaved persons stood in relation to free persons.

Mental diseases proven to be brain diseases cease to be psychiatric illnesses and become neurological illnesses—just as manumitted bondservants ceased to be slaves and became free persons. This is what happened to paresis, epilepsy, and Alzheimer's disease.

The table of contents of *Scientific American Medicine* (2001), section "Psychiatry," lists nine subsections, the subjects ranging from alcohol abuse and eating disorders to schizophrenia. Subsection V, titled "Alzheimer's Disease," is missing; instead, the following explanation appears in parentheses: "This subsection has been moved to Section 11 Neurology."[19]

* * *

Typically, bodily illness is something the patient *has,* mental illness, something he *does* or *is.*

* * *

Bodily illness is *in the patient's body*; mental illness is *in his record.*

* * *

A person is said to *get* a cold, *come down* with the flu, *develop* cancer; but he *goes* mad. The verb "goes" indicates that madness is a *doing,* not a *happening.*

* * *

Commitment laws invariably refer to the mental patient's "dangerousness to himself and/or others," illustrating that, ontologically, mental illness is something the person *does*, to himself or others.

* * *

We regularly read about "escaped mental patients" murdering people.

We never read about "escaped diabetes patients" committing such crimes.

Ergo: "Mental illness is like any other illness."

* * *

Doubt is to certainty as neurosis is to psychosis.

The neurotic is in doubt and has fears about persons and things.

The psychotic has convictions and makes claims about them.

The neurotic is disturbed, the psychotic is disturbing.

The neurotic has problems, the psychotic has solutions.

* * *

Psychiatric diagnoses are stigmatizing labels phrased to resemble medical diagnoses, applied to persons whose behavior annoys or offends others.

Persons who suffer from and complain of their own behavior are usually classified as neurotic.

Persons whose behavior makes others suffer, and about whom others complain, are usually classified as psychotic.

* * *

Webster's defines delusion as "something that is falsely or delusively believed..."

The *New Yorker* reports: "Last year, a Gallup poll found that half of all Americans believe in E.S.P. [extra-sensory perception], more than forty percent believe in demonic possession and haunted houses, and about a third believe in astrology, clairvoyance, and ghosts.... When I asked an Indian skeptic what problems his country was facing, he chuckled. 'Problems? In India, there are always problems,' he said. 'Right now, we have too many godmen. There are men who say they are gods. We have hundreds, thousands...'"[20]

* * *

Delusion of grandeur: Attributing cosmic significance to one's ordinary insignificance; self-aggrandizement by self-deception of goodness.

Delusion of worthlessness: Attributing cosmic insignificance to one's ordinary significance; self-aggrandizement by self-deception of badness.

* * *

Sartre said hysteria is a lie without a liar.[21] He could also have said that the hysteric is a liar who does not admit or recognize his lies.

* * *

Formerly, psychiatrists looked for the reason that the patient is depressed, and claimed that insight is therapeutic for it.

Now, psychiatrists assert that the patient has no reason to be depressed and claim that drugs are therapeutic for it.

What has remained constant is the *a priori* exclusion of the possibility that "it" is not a disease.

* * *

An old person suffering from a degenerative brain disease, such as Alzheimer's dementia, is like a fine building: once a comfortable home for families that has fallen into hopeless disrepair.

A young person suffering from "severe" mental disease, such as schizophrenia, is like an empty lot, for which a fine building was planned but never built.

* * *

What we call a mental illness, especially in a legal context, is a strategy, not a fact; a policy, not a disease.

* * *

If a man lies about his car so he that can get more money for it, that is economic behavior.

If he lies about himself so that he can get more attention, that is madness. We respond to one deception by bargaining about price, to the other by treating mental illness.

* * *

Virtually every bodily illness a person can have—cancer, pneumonia, myocardial infarction—a cadaver too can have.

But a cadaver cannot have a mental illness.

Nevertheless, it is the official position of the American Medical Association, the American Psychiatric Association, and the American state that "mental illness is like any other illness."

* * *

According to the classic, Virchowian definition, disease is an objective condition—the *patho-anatomical* or *pathophysiological* alteration of the body. At the beginning of the twentieth century, the category called "disease" was expanded to include *psychopathological* conditions of the mind, called "mental diseases," as diseases on a par with bodily diseases.

According to the classic, Christian definition, marriage is a formally recognized social institution—the legal and sexual union of a man and a woman. At the end of the twentieth century (in some Western countries), the category called "marriage" was expanded to include homosexual marriages as marriages on a par with heterosexual marriages.

There is nothing mysterious about such category-creep. The important thing to keep in mind is that it is not based on—in fact has nothing to do with—new discoveries, new knowledge, or science. Instead, it is based on and is motivated by ideological, legal, economic, moral, and political interests.

* * *

According to contemporary scientific psychiatry, there are two kinds of mental diseases: those whose neuropathological character has *already* been satisfactorily demonstrated, and those whose neuropathological character has *not yet* been so demonstrated.

The former are called "neurological diseases" and are treated by neurologists. The latter are called "psychiatric disorders" and are treated by psychiatrists.

This view now constitutes both scientific dogma and popular belief. The possibility that some terms used as psychiatric diagnoses do not name diseases is, *a priori,* ruled out of court.

* * *

Psychiatrists claim that mental diseases are caused by, or are the manifestations of, underlying bodily diseases.

If this were or proved to be true for some or all mental diseases, it would only add more items to the existing list of organic diseases whose treatment patients are free to reject. Hence, evidence supporting the organic etiology of so-called mental illness would display rather than dispel the moral and political dilemmas of coercive psychiatry.

* * *

Mental illness is (said to be a) brain disease that cannot be identified/diagnosed by biological markers. Instead, it is identified by its power to annul the criminal-law consequences of the actor's dramatically destructive behavior, for example, mass murder, without annulling the civil-law consequences of his dramatically creative behavior, for example, composing a great symphony.

* * *

Voyeurism is not an eye disease. Violence is not a brain disease.

* * *

When a healthy young person fails in life, we often say he is mentally ill. He fails because he is too conceited, too lazy, too stubborn, or lacks courage—explanations we are forbidden to entertain or articulate.

* * *

When an intelligent, physically healthy, well-educated young man from a comfortable family drops out of college and cannot make a go of his life, the politically correct assumption is that "there is something wrong with him," that the cause is mental illness, and that the alleged illness is a subtle type of brain disease best treated with mental hospitalization and neuroleptic drugs. This entire set of beliefs rests on the false assumption that failure to cope with life is a disease.

* * *

Calling a person mentally ill requires that he be existentially weak. Children, poor adults, and feeble old persons don't have the power to reject being cast in the role of mental patient.

Powerful persons cannot be cast in the role of mental patient, except by their enemies from far afar.

* * *

If mental diseases are brain diseases, then the relationship between mental patients and the state ought to be regulated by the same laws that regulate the relationship between neurological patients and the state. In practice, that would require that patients with paranoid schizophrenia and Parkinsonism be managed the same way with respect to competence, involuntary hospitalization, the right to reject treatment, and the insanity defense.

* * *

Seeing signs of mental illness in the brain is like seeing signs of bleeding in the Eucharistic host.[22] Biased premise, biased inference.

* * *

Every claim of a successful treatment of mental illness with a somatic intervention—electroshock, lobotomy, drugs—has been, at best, a claim for the efficacy of a type of faith healing or, at worst, a claim for the mutilation, as " treatment," of the patient's cognitive capacity to produce "mental symptoms."

Pickpocketing can be cured by cutting off the thief's hands. Its success, however, does not prove that theft is a bodily disease due to having hands, or that amputating hands is a treatment for it. It proves only that one needs hands to pick people's pockets.

* * *

The speed of light and the malignancy of melanoma are natural phenomena, discovered by scientists.

Speeding and schizophrenia are violations of behavioral rules mandated by politicians and psychiatrists.

* * *

If disease is defined as lesion, misbehavior cannot be disease. Psychiatrists overcome this obstacle by making use of the following four interpretations of the (mis)behavior of the non-sick person (NSP):

1. The NSP produces pain not attributable to a bodily source; the psychiatrist calls this "hysteria."

2. The NSP produces a self-induced lesion, such as urine he has deliberately bloodied; the psychiatrist calls this "factitious disorder" or "Munchausen syndrome."

3. NSP poisons another person, usually her own child; the psychiatrist calls this "Munchausen syndrome by proxy."

4. The NSP kills himself; the psychiatrist calls this the "fatal result of the untreated disease, depression."

* * *

The libertarian-philosophical commitment to the principle of self-ownership and to the prohibition against initiating violence is incompatible with the coercive practices of psychiatry. Nevertheless, many libertarians appear to believe in "mental illness." Hence, I shall briefly restate the basis for my objection to this concept, from a specifically libertarian point of view.

The term "mental illness" may or may not refer to an overt act. Kleptomania refers to an act—stealing—and the subject's claim that he cannot help it. Depression does not refer to an act; it refers to a "mental state." (Indeed, many persons diagnosed as depressed say they are not; that intensifies the psychiatrist's diagnostic zeal, who then adds that the "patient denies his illness.")

The libertarian principle of not initiating violence—combined with a belief in punishing persons who deprive others of life, liberty, or property—renders mental illness irrelevant. If the term refers to a crime, then the criminal ought to be punished. If the term refers to a "mental state" (and a presumed "dangerousness to self and others"), the person (called "mental patient") ought to be left unmolested by agents of the coercive apparatus of the state. Since psychologists and psychiatrists are legally and professionally obligated to deprive "seriously mentally ill" persons of liberty, they cannot be both libertarians and mental health professionals.

"Ideas," Richard Weaver cautioned, "have consequences." Hence, so, too, have the words that express ideas. The term "heretic" is harmless, when uttered by a layperson in America. It is not harmless, when uttered by a Muslim cleric in Saudi Arabia. Similarly, the term mental illness is not likely to have (serious) consequences, when pronounced by a layperson. However, it has far-reaching consequences, when "diagnosed" by a psychologist or psychiatrist, especially in a legal setting.

Using the term "mental illness"—without explicitly repudiating its consequences in civil commitment, in the insanity defense, and, last but not least, in contemporary American tort litigation, exemplified by the tobacco suits—is a betrayal of libertarian principles.

* * *

Scientists who try to prove the reality of mental illnesses by examining the brain make the same mistake as theologians who try to prove the divinity of Jesus by examining the Shroud of Turin.

A materialist explanation for "mental illnesses" would put an end to their being viewed as *mental* illnesses, exactly as a materialist explanation for "miracles" would put an end to their being viewed as miracles.

* * *

For the psychiatrist, mental illness is a problem (illness); for the patient, it is a solution (lifestyle); for the family, it is a moral excuse from badness; for the law, it is a legal excuse from crime; for the neuroscientist, it is an explanation of how the brain works; for the pharmaceutical company, it is a market for drugs; for the media, it is a source of sensational news.

* * *

The drug treatment of mental illness: psychiatrists prescribing drugs about which they know nothing, to patients about whom they know less.

* * *

The phenomena we now call "mental illnesses" are complex combinations of tragedy and troublemaking, displayed as diseases or so interpreted by others.

* * *

God and mental illness are powerful explanatory images/metaphors.

God cannot show his face, lest he be recognized as natural rather than supernatural and hence not God.

Mental illness cannot show its face, lest it be recognized as (mis)behavior and hence not disease.

* * *

Most people believe: 1) that the term "mental illness" names an objectively identifiable entity; and 2) that mental illnesses, such as depression and schizophrenia, belong in the same taxonomic class as do bodily illnesses, such as diabetes and uremia, because they are, in fact, diseases of the brain.

These beliefs are unshakeable because people accept as evidence: 1) that drugs are effective treatments for mental illnesses; 2) that "studies" about the relative efficacy of pharmacological and psychological therapy for mental illnesses prove that mental illnesses "exist" and are diseases; and 3) that "mental processes" are reducible to brain processes, in other words, that abnormal thinking is due to abnormal brain activity. For example, Lewis Wolpert, an eminent British embryologist, explains:

> If we understood how genes predispose to depression, it might be possible to design more effective drugs. Instead of criticizing the drug companies for trying to make money, we should be grateful for their antidepressants. We should not deny our biology when it comes to mental processes, whether normal or abnormal, *for every thought and feeling is the result of the activities of nerve cells in our brains.*[24]

* * *

Since psychotropic drugs have been declared to be effective treatments for mental diseases, psychiatrists have been "proving" that problems of living are real diseases by trotting out trophy patients—Kay Redfield Jamison, William Styron, Mike Wallace—who offer testimonials about how drugs saved their lives.

This tactic makes cures by psychiatry resemble cures at Lourdes. Yet, instead of diminishing the medical-scientific status of psychiatry, it enhances it.

* * *

Ignaz Semmelweis denied the medical doctrine that puerperal fever was due to "miasma"; he maintained that it was due to infection caused by the dirty hands of doctors.

I deny the medical doctrine that mental illness is due to chemical imbalance in the brain; I maintain that it is due to confusion caused by the dirty mouths of doctors.

* * *

Psychiatrists, first ladies, pharmaceutical companies, and lay members of mental health lobbies, such as NAMI (National Alliance for the Mentally Ill) never tire of telling the government, the media, and the public that mental illnesses are brain diseases.

When a board certified neurologist tries to testify in a commitment hearing about the mental illness of a person held for eleven years, the judge does not permit him to do so: "Circuit Judge William Schuwerk [in Chester, Illinois] said he would not allow such testimony [that there is no mental illness] because it was 'outside the general beliefs of the scientific community.'"[25]

* * *

All treatment entails a risk to the patient's health.

In the case of unforced medical treatment—for example, the use of female sex hormones for menopause—the patient is the ultimate arbiter of whether the benefits outweigh the risks.

In the case of forced psychiatric treatment—for example, the use of neuroleptic drugs for "severe mental illness"—the judge is the ultimate arbiter of whether the benefits outweigh the risks, even if the patient is legally competent.

* * *

Freud said the hysteric suffers from reminiscences. Not so. The hysteric suffers from his inability or unwillingness to come to terms with his memories. The psychiatrist legitimizes this evasion, transforming it into an illness—and a mystery, that only he can unravel.

The psychotic, too, could be said to suffer from reminiscences. Once again, it would be more accurate to say that he suffers from his inability or unwillingness to come to terms with his memories, exemplified by Lady Macbeth. The psychiatrist legitimizes the patient's evasion by transforming it into a serious illness—a mysterious brain disorder that only he can cure.

In this sense, mental illness is a result of a collusion between the individual, *qua* mental patient, and the psychiatrist, *qua* medical mystery worker. The "doctor" transforms the "patient" from a person *qua* agent plagued by memories, into a body *qua* receptacle plagued by lesions.

* * *

The paranoid is a person who insists you don't like him, when in fact you don't, but when the polite thing for him to do would be to keep quiet about it.

* * *

There are two radically different types of "mental patients." Some are inadequate, unskilled, lazy, or stupid persons. Others are gifted persons, protesters, revolutionaries, or individuals on strike against their relatives and society.

Because psychiatrists do not differentiate between the unfit and the unwilling, they often attribute unfitness to unwillingness, and unwillingness to unfitness.

* * *

If a person doesn't listen to his inner voice when young, he may, before long, find himself "hearing voices" that he'll think come from without.

* * *

The tyrant forces people to be unfree. The insane person forces people to treat him as if he were unfree.

The tyrant terrorizes by means of naked power; the psychotic, by means of the brutal drama of madness.

The tyrant plays shepherd, forcing people to be sheep; the psychotic plays lost sheep, forcing people to be his shepherd.

* * *

Long ago, two great Englishmen told us—much better than modern psychiatrists tell us—what "mental illness" is.

> Thomas Hobbes, 1651: "The passion, whose violence, or continuance, maketh madness, is either great vainglory; which is commonly called *pride*, and *self-conceit*; or great *dejection* of mind.... In sum, all passions that produce strange and unusual behaviour, are called by the general name of madness."[26]

> Samuel Butler, 1882: "All our lives long, every day and every hour, we are engaged in the process of accommodating our changed and unchanged selves to changed and unchanged surroundings, living, in fact, is nothing else than this process of accommodation; when we fail in it a little we are stupid, when we fail flagrantly we are mad, when we suspend it temporarily we sleep, when we give up the attempt altogether we die."[27]

* * *

In recent decades, the mental health industry has spawned a new specialist: the critic of therapy. His self-appointed role is to condemn drug treatment, or psychotherapy, or both, without acknowledging that there is no mental illness.

By selectively criticizing the *treatment of mental illness*, he validates its reality.[28] (See also *Madness*)

Mental Patients

Many former mental patients call themselves "psychiatric survivors" or "consumers of mental health services." They deny that "mental illnesses" are diseases, but affirm that they are disabled by it, deserve to be supported by disability payments for mental illness, and ought to receive, gratis, "mental health services" whose nature and distribution they define and control.

Liberated slaves did not want or expect to receive "plantation services" from their former masters. Yet, that is exactly what many liberated psychiatric slaves expect and demand to receive from the psychiatrists and the state that enslaved them. Unfortunately, many self-styled critics of psychiatry support that absurd expectation and demand.

Message/Messenger

In debates about contentious social policies, it's the institutional prestige of the messenger that counts, not the contents of the message.

The nonsensical views of a "Princeton philosopher" command respectful attention. The sensible views of a "Podunk philosopher" are ignored.

Perhaps it was always thus. Now, when media attention defines merit, it is especially so.

Mind

Mind is a verb.

Somatic treatments of mental illness—lobotomy, electroshock, and psychotropic drugs—impair the person's ability to mind. Since the mental patient is viewed—by himself and/or others—as a person who minds the wrong things, his diminished capacity to mind is deemed to be an improvement of his illness.

* * *

The telephone does not explain how we speak, or the computer, how we think.

The PET scan cannot explain what is in our mind.

Calling the mind the "brain" is like burning a book and calling the ashes its "content."

* * *

As long as a person is alive and conscious, his mind minds, just as his heart beats and his kidneys secrete urine.

If the mind has nothing to mind outside of itself, it tries to obliterate itself, with drugs, noise, sex, and mental illness.

Money

He who pays the piper calls the tune.

* * *

People value what they pay for, and pay for what they value.

* * *

Money talks. But only the greedy and gullible listen.

Monomedicine

Monomedicine is the worship of a single, legitimate system of diagnosing and treating disease, authorized by the state to enforce its practice and in turn legitimizing the state as therapeutic: the therapeutic state.

Monomedicine resembles and reprises monotheism as the worship of a single, legitimate system of recognizing and worshiping God, authorized by the state to enforce its practice and in turn legitimizing the state as theological: the theological state.

We reject and guard against the alliance of the state with a monopoly on the legitimate use of force and religion. But we embrace and cultivate the alliance of the state with a monopoly on the legitimate use of force and medicine.

We have tragically misinterpreted the nature, and overestimated the extent, of personal freedom and individual responsibility we have gained since the Scientific Revolution.

* * *

The theological state represented a "monoconfessional" community.[29]
The therapeutic state represents a "monomedical" community.

* * *

Monotheistic religions tranquilize people with heaven, and terrify them with hell.

Monomedical "religions" do the same thing with drugs. (See also *Therapeutic State*)

Morals

Formerly, people thanked God for the good in their life and blamed themselves for the evil in it.

Today, people take credit for the good in their life and blame others for the evil in it, whom they then proceed to sue for damages. (See also *Ethics*)

Mystery

Only a person unable to see the mystery of the natural world finds mystery in the supernatural world.

Myth of Mental Illness

Bodily illness is to mental illness as literal meaning is to metaphorical meaning.

* * *

Looking for the organic etiology of mental illness is like looking for the caloric content of food for thought.

* * *

Treating mental illness with brain surgery, electricity passed through the head, or chemicals is about as sensible and effective as trying to keep warm by burning the family tree.

* * *

Mental illness is a myth whose function is to disguise and thus render more palatable the bitter pill of moral conflicts in human relations. In asserting that there is no such thing as mental illness I do not deny that people have problems coping with life and each other.

* * *

We may be dissatisfied with television for two quite different reasons: because our set does not work, or because we dislike the program we are receiving. Similarly, we may be dissatisfied with ourselves for two quite different reasons: because our body does not work (bodily illness), or because we dislike our conduct (mental illness).

It is foolish to try get rid of beer commercials by having TV repairmen work on our sets. It is just as foolish to try to get rid of phobias, obsessions, and delusions by having psychiatrists work on our brains.

* * *

In 1960, I proposed the phrase "myth of mental illness" to emphasize that the phenomena we call "mental illnesses" are neither mental nor illnesses, that the persons we call "mental patients" are not ill, and that the measures used to remedy these alleged diseases are not treatments but efforts to tranquilize, pacify, and subdue the disturbed or, more often, the disturbing person.[30]

* * *

The bat flies through the air and looks like a bird—but is not a bird.
The whale swims in water and looks like a fish—but is not a fish.
The koala looks like a bear—but is not a bear.
Mental illnesses may look like diseases—but are not diseases.

* * *

Cancer and diabetes are literal diseases: no one doubts that they are diseases of body or ignores their somatic basis.

Lovesickness and homesickness are metaphorical diseases: no one (yet) claims that they are diseases of the body and looks for their somatic basis.

Where do mental illnesses belong? Are they literal or metaphorical illnesses?

It seems remarkable that simply because they have names such as "schizophrenia" and "bipolar illness," psychiatrists, politicians, journalists, and people in general feel certain that these terms refer to brain diseases and look for their somatic basis in the chemistry of nerve cells.

* * *

It is springtime. A student visits a psychiatrist. His complaint is that he feels bored, lethargic, unable to study. The psychiatrist makes a diagnosis of "spring fever" and prescribes a drug. Soon the patient reports that he feels better and is functioning better. Ergo, spring fever is a disease.

A mother brings her son, in the springtime of his life, to a psychiatrist. Her complaint is that he has dropped out of college, shows no interest in doing anything useful, stays up at night and smokes marijuana. The psychiatrist makes a diagnosis of "schizophrenia" and prescribes a drug. Soon the mother reports that her son feels better and behaves better.

Ergo, schizophrenia is a disease.

* * *

When a physician restores the life of a person whose heart has stopped, he proves that it is possible to *revive* moribund persons, not that it is possible to *resurrect* the dead.

Were a psychiatrist to discover that a mental patient suffers from a brain disease, he would prove that persons called "mental patients" may have brain diseases, not that mental diseases are brain diseases.

* * *

We think that identifying a person as mentally ill is like identifying him as hypertensive; in fact, it is more like identifying him as ugly.

Although there may be widespread agreement among members of a particular group or society with the "diagnosis," there is nothing objective or objectifiable about it, comparable, say, to a blood count or blood pressure measurement.

* * *

The patient with bodily illness, experiencing suffering, is driven to see a physician by pain.

The patient with mental illness, making others suffer, is driven to see a psychiatrist by the police.

The difference between bodily illness and mental illness is like the difference between the ways the word *driven* is used in these two sentences.

* * *

Literal diseases—such as malaria or melanoma—deprive the patient of life *without* the additional help of human agency: pathogenic microorganisms or tumor cells kill him.

Metaphorical diseases—such as clinical depression and schizophrenia—deprive the patient of life only *with* the help of human agency: the patient kills himself or another person or persons kill him.

* * *

The Greeks and the Romans had many gods. The Jews had only one.

Dissatisfied with monotheism, some Jews must have longed for at least one additional deity, more real than their invisible and unportrayable god. They invented Jesus, the Son of God, a ready literalization of the then common metaphoric phrase, "son of God."

We have only one conception of disease: bodily abnormality.

Dissatisfied with the monocriterial, monomedical conception of disease, we long for additional diseases. We invent mental disease, a ready literalization of the common metaphoric phrase, "it's a sickness."

Thus, we convert unwanted behaviors into diseases and, instead of worshiping many gods, worship the search for new treatments for the hundreds of mental diseases that ail us.

* * *

In 1988, the United States Office of Patents and Trademarks placed its imprimatur on the literalization of the metaphor of mental illness. In the case of *Stacy v. Jones*, it stated: "A chemical that can be injected into the body and scanned with X-rays for diagnosis of mental disease has been invented by two Georgetown University professors.... Patent 4,716,225, granted this week, is assigned to the university.... Schizophrenia and manic-depression are among the ailments that can be detected with the method."[31]

* * *

If a person does not believe in God or heaven, he is a hypocrite if he claims that prayer is ineffective for facilitating the trip to heaven.

Similarly, if a person does not believe in mental illness or psychiatric treatment, he is a hypocrite if he claims that antipsychotic drugs are ineffective for treating mental illness.

* * *

More than forty years have passed since I first suggested that there is, and can be, no such thing as mental illness.

Since then, with great fanfare, psychiatrists have announced that this or that mental illness—for example, homosexuality, hysteria, neurosis itself—is not a mental illness.

Such claims attract much popular attention, perhaps because they simultaneously assert and deny the validity of the concept of mental illness. *By asserting that X is not a mental illness, the experts imply that Y and Z are.*

Formerly, people wanted both to believe and disbelieve in the existence of witches. Now, they want both to believe and disbelieve in the existence of mental illness.

* * *

My suggestion that mental illness is not a disease was immediately and instinctively viewed as an attempt to redistribute the profits from madness, as if I were proposing taking it away from psychiatrists and giving it to psychologists. I intended no such thing.

Referring to so-called mental illnesses as "problems in living" or "personal problems" does not imply that these phenomena are the property of any profession or group of professionals. I have steadfastly emphasized that the issue of the ownership of personal conduct—healthy or sick, sane or insane—is an integral part of the problem of so-called mental illness; and that, if we wish to come to grips with this problem, we must decide whether we value freedom more highly than health, or vice versa.

I value freedom more highly than health and advocate returning diseases and mental diseases to their rightful owners, medical patients and mental patients.

* * *

One of the arguments against my claim that there is no mental illness has hardened into a dogma that seems to convince most people that I must be wrong. It goes like this: "We believe in the medical approach to mental illness. There are others—they may or may not mention me by name—who prefer the social approach to it. But they are wrong, because..." Then they then cite studies about the genetics of schizophrenia, or x-ray studies of the brains of schizophrenics, or the effectiveness of drugs for controlling "it."

I am frequently confronted with this argument, especially by reporters. I have concluded that it is founded on so successful a distortion of my position that it is virtually impossible to counter it. If a well-intentioned questioner does not see the point on which this riddle turns, no amount of fresh explanation about the mythology of mental illness is likely to make him see it. Still, I try to answer it, along this line:

> Let us go back four hundred years. People then believed in witches and the Inquisition. Suppose someone had come along and said: "There are no

> witches; the term 'witch' is merely a name we attach to some poor and helpless people, usually women, persecuted by the Inquisition." Would it be proper to call this person's position on witches a "social approach" to witchcraft, as opposed to a "theological approach" to it? Of course not. What this person offers is not a sociological approach to witches, but a philosophical criticism of the people who call other people "witches" and persecute them on that basis.

Everyone now knows that witches don't exist, and that mental diseases do.

* * *

My critics say that I "deny the reality of mental illness," and cannot understand why I do not consider this an acceptable summary of my view.

Would they consider it an acceptable summary of their view to say that they share the "delusion that mental illness is like any other illness"?

* * *

A person planning to become an exorcist could not be expected to show much interest in the proposition that demonic possession is a myth. Faced with the possibility of the non-existence of possession, he would feel compelled to dismiss either the idea that possession is a myth or his plan to become an exorcist.

Mutatis mutandis, a person planning to become a psychiatrist cannot be expected to show much interest in the proposition that mental illness is a myth. Faced with the possibility of the non-existence of mental illness, he would feel compelled to dismiss either the idea that mental illness is a myth or his plan to become a psychiatrist.

Similar considerations apply to the person who seeks to consult an exorcist or psychiatrist. If there is no demonic possession, one cannot be exorcized of demons. If there is no mental illness, one cannot be cured of it.

Although many people feel, in their hearts, that there is no mental illness, few believe, in their heads, that they can afford to act as if that were true.

* * *

For the past forty-five years, one psychiatrist after another has dismissed my books, asserting that I repeat my "one good idea," that mental illness is a myth. But if that is such a good idea, why don't psychiatrists accept it as valid?

* * *

Hearing me say that I don't believe in mental illness, people invariably ask: "How, then, can you be a professor of psychiatry?"

I reply: "The same way that a person who does not believe in God can be a professor of religion. Such a person studies the history of various religions and the behavior of persons who believe in them; teaches about diverse religions and their particular claims and rules; and writes about his own reflections on the subject. That is what I do with respect to mental illness and psychiatry."

* * *

Having listened to my criticism of psychiatry, people often ask, "Well, what do you replace it with? What do you propose we do with mental patients?"

Although I am mindful of the wisdom of Jonathan Swift's remark that, "It is useless to attempt to reason a man out of a thing he was never reasoned into," politeness dictates that I answer:

- Imagine that you live in western Europe in the sixteenth century and believe there are no witches and oppose burning them at the stake. You are asked: "Well, what do you suggest we do with the witches?" You would answer: "Stop burning them."

- Imagine that you live in Alabama in 1850 and are an abolitionist. You are asked, "Well, what do suggest we do with slaves?" You would answer: "Stop enslaving them."

If someone wants to *help* a so-called mental patient, the first thing he must do is eschew coercing him. The next thing he can do is help the person on his terms or leave him alone.

* * *

"The poet's pen gives to airy nothing...a name," wrote Shakespeare.[32]
The priest's pen gives to certain revered persons a name—*saint.*
The psychiatrist's pen gives to certain rejected people a name—*mentally ill.*

Everyone's speech engages in this kind of naming, with the result that, in Robert Reininger's (German philosopher, 1869-1955) words: "*Unser Weltbild ist immer zugleich ein Wertbild*" (Our view of the world is, at the same time, a view of [our] values).[33]

Sainthood and mental illness are both fictions, that is, fabricated products. One is manufactured by authoritative rhetorical acts of *benediction*, the other by authoritative rhetorical acts of *malediction.*

The pretense that creating a new psychiatric diagnosis is an act of *discovering* a disease—that inventing a name is discovering a phenomenon, that a rhetorical trick is an empirical finding—underlies the entire apparatus of psychiatric nosology.

* * *

I coined the phrase "myth of mental illness" to identify my unqualified rejection of the psychiatric belief in mental illness as an objectively identifiable phenomenon, cause, and explanation.

Many so-called critics of psychiatry say this is an overstatement—for example, that attention deficit disorder (ADD) is not a mental illness, but schizophrenia is. This is like a modern, scientifically enlightened person's use of God-language. Faced with the tragedy of a village virtually destroyed by a landslide, he recoils from saying that God caused the catastrophe killing thousands, but may readily say that God saved the few who survived.

A person cannot claim be to a critic of religious mythology without denying the core beliefs of religion, such as the divinity of Jesus.

A person cannot claim to be a critic of psychiatric mythology without denying the disease status of mental illness.

As God is never a cause and explanation of natural events, mental illness is never a cause or explanation of human behavior.

* * *

The power of an idea whose time has come is said to be irresistible. Today, mental illness is such an idea.

This is why I believe that the problem with psychiatry is not so much that psychiatrists have too much power, although they do. It is rather that the idea of mental illness has too much power, given to it by the people who believe in it.

Only when people relinquish their blind faith in mental health and mental illness will they see fit to curb the powers of psychiatry, just as only when people abandoned their blind faith in God and the Devil did they see fit to curb the powers of priestcraft.

The kind of power psychiatrists now wield is similar to the kind of power priests wielded before the Enlightenment. It does not come out of the barrel of a gun held by an oppressor; it comes out of beliefs held by human beings who prefer to rely on mystifying symbols and paternalistic authorities rather than on themselves.

* * *

We owe to Immanuel Kant the important distinction between what he called "analytic truths" and "synthetic truths."

- We know the truth of an analytic proposition if we know the meanings of the words involved: we know that bachelors are unmarried without having to investigate their marital status. We know the truth of a synthetic proposition by its relation to facts in the world: we know that the capital of New York State is Albany by reference to appropriate records.

- In an analytic proposition, the predicate is contained in the subject. In a synthetic proposition, the predicate cannot be arrived at by an analysis of the terms employed.

- *Analytic truths are "truths of reason": they result from reasoning and the precise use of language. Synthetic truths are "truths of fact": they result from experience of the world.*

- We need rationalist methods to verify analytic statements, empirical methods to verify synthetic statements.

When, in 1960, I first asserted that mental illness is a myth, I meant to remind people that, according to strict medical definition, disease is a predicate of *(human) bodies.* If we grant that definition, then we need not examine any particular person to know that he does not have a *mental illness*. The mind can be ill only in a metaphorical sense. Why is this simple proposition so difficult to accept and why is it so often misunderstood and misrepresented? Three reasons spring to mind:

1. A person "diagnosed" as ill—that is, said to have a disease or believed to have a disease—may or may not have a disease. We cannot know whether the statement "John Doe has acute appendicitis" is true or false without examining him. And even if we examine him, our conclusion

that he does not have appendicitis may be erroneous. People assume that the same considerations apply to the person suspected of being mentally ill.

2. My claim that mental illness is a myth, albeit cognitively obvious, is linguistically obscure. The claim re-asserts an analytic truth that people perceive as if it were a synthetic truth, subject to falsification by means of empirical observation. The claim is misunderstood, as well, because people, especially educated people, equate mental disease with brain disease. Psychiatry is a branch of medicine. Psychiatrists and other authorities regularly assert that mental diseases are brain diseases. Thus, when a "normal" person hears me say that there is no such thing as mental illness, he is likely to counter: "But I know persons who were diagnosed as mentally ill and have turned out to have X (neurosyphilis, multiple sclerosis, brain tumor). In due time, with refinements in medical technology, psychiatrists will be able to show that all mental illnesses are bodily diseases."

   The example of the bachelor as an unmarried person may clarify this fashionable conundrum. Suppose that my interlocutor were to misinterpret this definition, which asserts an analytic truth, as if it were a synthetic truth. He might then reply: "But I know several bachelors who were secretly married. Hence, there are married bachelors." This is fallacious. There may well be persons in the world who claim to be bachelors, or whom others believe to be bachelors, who in fact are married. But regardless of how many such persons there may be in the world, the word "bachelor" denotes an unmarried person.

   Trying to prove the *existence of mental illnesses*, psychiatric loyalists often engage in precisely such a tactic: they look for married bachelors, in an effort to prove that the word "bachelor" does not mean unmarried person; that is, they look for abnormalities in the brain to prove that mental illness does not mean disease of the mind. The believer in psychiatric miracles has replaced the believer in religious miracles: seeing signs of mental illness in the brain is like seeing signs of bleeding in the Eucharistic host.[34]

   Undoubtedly, there are persons who claim to be, or whom others believe to be, mentally ill who have a disease of the brain or some other part of the body. My critics conclude that this proves that mental illnesses are genuine diseases. This is fallacious. If a person has a disease of the brain or some other organ, then he has a neurological illness or some other disease, not a mental illness. Regardless of how many such persons there may be in the world, the word "disease" denotes a condition of the body.

3. The third reason for misunderstanding and misrepresenting the meaning of my claim that mental illness is a myth is, broadly speaking, existential. For psychiatrists, abandoning the idea of mental illness would require and entail relinquishing the advantages that society bestows on persons it credits with medical authority; for lay persons, it would require and entail relinquishing the resources that the mental health industry offers in dealing with their personal problems and the personal problems of their relatives.

Religious symbolism is saturated with what believers view as miracles, and what non-believers regard as oxymorons, literalized metaphors, or deceptions and self-deceptions. A Catholic priest cannot deny the miracle of transubstantiation and remain a priest. In the religion of "mental health," a psychiatric diagnosis of mental illness—homosexuality, smoking marijuana, hearing voices—is miraculously transformed into a disease of the brain. The psychiatrist who "denies" this miracle is not only cast out of the profession, his views are ignored as uninformed criticisms of psychiatry unworthy of attention. It is small wonder that very few psychiatrists have taken that step.

N

Nationalism

Nationalism trumps rationalism.

Nature

We use mathematics to formulate the laws of physical nature, proverbs to formulate the laws of human nature.

Needs

Children get what their parents decide they *need*. Adults buy what they decide they *want*.

Statist medicine turns adults into children.

The government gives people *permission* to buy and use the drugs it decides they need, and *prohibits* them from buying or using the drugs people decide they want.

Popular acceptance of this paternalistic substitution of needs for wants—of medicalized permissions for personal decisions—is emblematic of how readily the American people have embraced medical statism, and rejected individual liberty and personal responsibility.

O

Old Age

Old age is when you begin to have less to say and talk more to strangers; when the quantity of your life becomes more important than its quality.

Organ Donation

The physicians who remove organs for transplantation; the technicians who test and preserve them; the persons who transport them; the hospitals where physicians transplant them; the physicians who transplant them; the pharmaceutical companies that manufacture the anti-rejection drugs without which the transplanted organs are useless; the pharmacists who sell the anti-rejection drugs; the medical ethicists who pontificate about the ethics of organ donation—all these persons get paid for their services.

Only the person who donates the organ—the linchpin in the chain of organ donation who makes all this possible—receives no payment for his own property, ostensibly *on moral grounds.*

Why? Because if he were paid, he—not the experts—would be the most important person in the enterprise.

Other, The

In the Age of Faith, the priest was not supposed to and was unable to see the Other as a person whose soul is none of his business; he could perceive him only as a morally defective sinner whom he must save from going to hell.

In the Age of Therapy, the psychiatrist is not supposed to and is unable to see the Other as a person whose mind is none of his business; he can perceive him only as a sick patient whom he must save from being a danger to himself or others.

P

Paranoid Schizophrenia

The paranoid schizophrenic is the person who craves recognition too eagerly and too impatiently: He is too ambitious, too energetic, too conceited; he cannot wait, work, and create the context in which his worth will be recognized by others.

By the time he reaches his late teens or early twenties, he feels the time has come for people to recognize him as the superior person he is. He becomes arrogant and haughty, overplays his hand, and plummets to earth, a human wreck. His craving for attention unfulfilled, he imagines that people are watching him, spying on him, harassing him: he is, once again, a *wunderkind*, the center of attention.

In short, paranoid schizophrenia is a kind of premature existential ejaculation. For a perfectly wrought illustration of this tragedy, see *A Beautiful Mind* by Sylvia Nasar.[1] (See also *Mental Illness*, *Psychiatry*)

Parents

One of the greatest challenges of being a parent is to encourage the child to be self-reliant, but not self-centered.

* * *

Formerly, parents unable to cope with their children enlisted relatives to help them or hired governesses and tutors. Now, they hire psychiatrists, psychologists, and mental hospitals.

* * *

Parents who cannot tolerate the unhappiness of their child will be compelled to endure his unhappiness as an adult.

* * *

The world would be a better place if parents valued their obligation to love and care for their children more highly than their obligation to love and care for each other.

A conflict between these obligations arises whenever the welfare of a child requires protecting him from the influences of a destructive father (husband) or mother (wife).

Paternalism

The paternalist says: "Do as I say." He wants disciples to indulge him and inflate his ego.

The individualist says: "Do as I do." He wants partners to talk to and learn from.

Patient Role

Being classified as ill may be advantageous or disadvantageous for the patient or for the doctor.

The questions that modern societies must face are: What should be our economic and legal attitude toward persons who classify themselves as ill, but are not? What should be our economic and legal attitude toward doctors who classify healthy persons as ill?

Pen

The pen, says the proverb, is mightier than the sword. This is but a partial truth.

In books and libraries, truth is more powerful than force. On the battlefield of everyday life, it is not.

The moral: Social criticism and political action do not mix. The true social critic cannot be an effective social activist, and vice versa.

Personal Conduct

A glossary:

Anxiety: The unwillingness to play even when the odds are for you.

Boredom: The feeling that everything is a waste of time.

Courage: The willingness to play even when the odds are against you.

Greatness: The willingness to expose one's littleness and risk embarrassment.

Happiness: An imaginary condition, formerly attributed by the living to the dead, now by adults to children, and by children to adults.

Serenity: The feeling that all is well with the world.

* * *

Clear thinking requires courage rather than intelligence.

* * *

If you don't listen to yourself, you won't hear what others say.

* * *

You don't have to be healthy to be happy.

* * *

We gain knowledge by learning, trust by doubt, skill by practice, and love by love.

* * *

The stupid neither forgive nor forget; the naive forgive and forget; the wise forgive but do not forget.

* * *

People often say that this or that person has not yet found himself. But the self is not something one finds; it is something one creates.

* * *

One of the most important motives for personal conduct is the desire to avoid boredom. To satisfy this need, people turn to food and drink, sex and work, crime and conquest.

* * *

The proverb warns that you should not bite the hand that feeds you. But if the hand prevents you from feeding yourself, that's exactly what you must do.

* * *

Men are often afraid to rock the boat in which they hope to drift safely through life's dangerous currents, when, in fact, the boat is stuck on a sandbar.

They would be better off to rock the boat and try to shake it loose or, better still, jump in the water and swim for the shore.

* * *

A good life requires that we learn not only to acquire habits but also to break habits.

* * *

Some disabled persons dwell on what they have lost, others focus on what they have left.

The former use their limitations as an excuse for parasitism, the latter, as an incentive for productivity.

* * *

The person securely in control of himself frustrates others from controlling him; hence, he is the object of both admiration and envy, awe and hate.

* * *

The quacks who tout self-esteem peddle conceit, which they have in abundance.

* * *

The price of liberty is vigilance. *Mutatis mutandis*, the price of independence is self-determination; the price of dignity, self-assertion; and the price of respect, respect for others and self-respect.

* * *

Good digestion requires hydrochloric acid; good thinking, adrenaline.

* * *

If you have strongly held opinions, you are opinionated; if you don't, you lack conviction.

Either way, there is something wrong with you.

* * *

Impertinence: The name superiors give to the aspirations for independence of their inferiors.

* * *

In close personal relationships, people often either envy or pity one another. Both sentiments poison friendship.

* * *

Articulate persons argue. Inarticulate persons quarrel.

* * *

Beware of the person who treats you as if he has no obligations to you. Like a rapist, he will reduce you to an object of his desires—to satisfy his lust for self-gratification.

Beware of the person who treats you as if you have no obligations to him. Like a therapist, he will reduce you to an object of his duties—to satisfy his lust for self-esteem.

* * *

Men hate waiting, for a few hours, while their wives shop for clothes and trinkets.

Women hate waiting, often for much of their lives, while their husbands shop for fame and glory.

* * *

We spend much of our time making money or spending it. Only when we gamble, can we do both at once, the proportion varying with our luck.

* * *

Men diet to live longer; women, to look better.

* * *

Obesity is to eating as promiscuity is to sex. For the religious, both are sins; for the pharmacrat, diseases; for the libertarian, the unhealthy and unaesthetic consequences of over-exercising the fundamental human right to one's self.

* * *

Economists talk about booms and busts, psychiatrists about mania and melancholia.

Both phenomena are the manifestations of human nature in a state of freedom. *Unless properly constrained by self-discipline*, the market fluctuates between manic highs fueled by greed and melancholic lows fueled by fear, while the individual fluctuates between self-assured, self-indulgent overactivity and self-doubting, self-loathing underactivity.

* * *

A victim is a person injured by another, for example, a drunk driver.

Traditionally, a person injured by himself, for example, a drunkard, was regarded as a sinner, not a victim. Today, he too is categorized as a victim, of mental illness.

Traditionally, the metaphorical victim was punished doubly, by social sanctions imposed on him by others, and by the biological consequences of his behavior imposed on him by his own body. Today, regarded as a literal victim, he is compensated for sickness, not punished for wickedness.

In March 1988, a Federal District Court in Florida ruled that a federal employee "who drank a pint of gin a day [and] was dismissed from his job after missing...389 days of work [in three years]...was legally crippled by alcoholism." The judge ordered the agency "to give him more than $150,000 in back pay" and ordered that the former employee be allowed to reapply for his old job.[2]

* * *

Self-control and self-esteem vary directly: The more self-esteem a person has, the greater, as a rule, is his desire, and ability, to control himself.

The desire to control others and self-esteem vary inversely: The less self-esteem a person has, the greater is his desire, but not his ability, to control others.

* * *

"Where there is a will, there is a way," says the proverb. Not always true.

But it is always true that where there is no will, there is no way.

* * *

Philanthropic generosity: giving willingly what belongs to oneself and doing so selflessly, even anonymously. Typical of individualists and selfish capitalists.

Political compassion: coercing others to give what belongs to them, claiming credit for helping the needy, and compelling the beneficiaries to pay personal and political obeisance to the coercer. Typical of collectivists and selfless anti-capitalists.

* * *

Men cannot long survive without air, water, and sleep. Next in importance comes food. And close on its heels, solitude.

* * *

We need other people. This is why solitary confinement is a severe punishment.

We also need solitude. "Hell is other people," said Sartre. Sometimes, being confined with others is a greater punishment than being alone.

* * *

Formerly, men wanted to *do* a good job; from that desire arose craftsmanship.

Today, they *want* a good job; from that desire arise unions and affirmative action programs.

* * *

Sooner or later, every person must ask himself: What should I do with my life? What shall I make?

A person can make money, machines, food, works of art, children, and many other things.

The person who decides that he doesn't want to, or can't, make anything at all, can always fall back on making trouble—the product in which psychotics, psychiatrists, and politicians specialize.

* * *

The person who feels entrapped by life has three options: 1. He can kill himself. 2. He can kill someone else, compelling others to kill him or confine him. 3. He can go mad, engaging in behavior viewed as crazy, compelling others to care for him as a mental patient.

* * *

If a person does something we disapprove of, we regard him as bad if we believe persuasion or punishment will deter him from persisting in his conduct, and as mad if we believe that these methods will not be sufficient.

* * *

The four categories of persons who can be relied on not to keep promises: politicians, psychiatrists, psychopaths, and psychotics.

* * *

Psychiatrists and psychologists assert that in order to develop optimally, children need an optimal familial and social environment. This is not true.

Only plants and animals need an optimal environment for optimal development. Human beings do not. More often than not, optimal familial and social conditions stunt rather than stimulate the child's moral development.

To develop as persons, children need optimal obstacles and the ability to cope with them successfully. This enables them to become competent performers in life and responsible moral agents.

* * *

Most people want liberty and self-determination for themselves and subjection for others.

Some want subjection for everyone.

Few want liberty and self-determination for everyone.

* * *

The masochist's maxim: It is better to be wanted as a victim than not to be wanted at all.

* * *

You can't teach an old dog new tricks, but you can an old man. That's one of the differences between dog and man.

* * *

Success, people say, is not everything. Nothing is everything: No achievement, relationship, or possession can satisfy the restlessness of the human spirit.

* * *

The man who professes unwavering belief in God and conventional wisdom is respected as a pillar of society, even if his everyday behavior is vile.

The man who openly rejects God, religion, and conventional wisdom is distrusted as "godless" and therefore wicked, even if his everyday behavior is exemplary.

Pharmacracy

"Inasmuch as we have words to describe medicine as a healing art, but have none to describe it as a method of social control or political rule, we must first give it a name. I propose that we call it *pharmacracy*, from the Greek roots *pharmakon*, for 'medicine' or 'drug,' and *kratein,* for 'to rule' or 'to control.'... As theocracy is rule by God or priests, and democracy is rule by the people or the majority, so pharmacracy is rule by medicine or physicians."[3]

* * *

For almost two hundred years, the United States exemplified the virtues of religious tolerance: the American government resisted making religious observance the business of the state and refused to practice persecution in the name of God. Now, it exemplifies the wickedness of pharmacological intolerance: it makes the use of pharmaceutical agents the business of the state and practices persecution in the name of drugs and health.

History tells us that religious peace—letting each person decide which god, if any, to worship—is preferable to religious war. Common sense tells us that pharmacological peace—letting each person decide what drug, if any, to ingest, inhale, or inject—is preferable to pharmacological war.

Physician

The physician, like Janus, has two faces. One is that of the independent healer, serving the medical needs of his patient, as the patient sees his needs. The other is that of the soldier, serving the political needs of the state, as the rulers of the state see those needs.

The emblems of the private physician are the house call and the white coat: the willingness to render a personal service in the patient's home signifies humility; the medical uniform signifies professional status and presumed competence.

The emblems of the public physician are the surgeon general and the military uniform: the office suggests violence rather than healing; the Public Health uniform signifies political status and the authority to use the coercive power of the state.

Placebo

Physicians who claim that placebos are effective therapeutic agents ought to be anesthetized for major surgery with placebos instead of anesthetics, and treated for postoperative pain with placebos instead of analgesics.

Politeness

Politeness: one of the most neglected and underrated virtues of our age.

* * *

So-called mental patients are impolite more often than medical patients or healthy persons. Neither psychiatrists nor other observers of the human scene seem to have paid much attention to this fact.

Perhaps habitually impolite behavior predisposes the person to "developing mental illness," much as smoking predisposes him to developing lung cancer.

Political Correctness

C. S. Lewis:

> One passes to the realization that our own age is also a "period," and certainly has, like all periods, its own characteristic illusions. They are likeliest to lurk in those widespread assumptions which are so ingrained in the age that no one dares to attack or feels it necessary to defend them.[4]

Politics

The state: a factory, equipped with a monopoly on the legitimate use of force, fabricating falsehoods defined as truths.

* * *

Types of tyranny:

Economic: The authorities pauperize the people.

Political: The authorities enslave the people.

Psychiatric: The authorities invalidate the people.

* * *

In the days of the Founding Fathers, the elitists were egalitarians. They did not fear making their inferiors their equals: embracing the free market, they saw their inferiors as potential collaborators, rather than potential competitors.

Today, the elitists are paternalists. They fear making their inferiors their equals: rejecting the free market, they see their inferiors only as potential competitors.

* * *

The Ten Commandments is a set of restraints, directed at the individual: its aim is to domesticate personal passions by limiting the powers of the individual, resulting in persons fit to live in harmony in society.

The Bill of Rights—that is, the first ten Amendments to the Constitution—is a set of restraints directed at the government: its aim is to domesticate political passions by limiting the powers of the rulers, resulting in societies fit for persons who value individual liberty and personal responsibility.

The first set of restraints is necessary to make an individual a civilized person, the second set, to make a society a civilized polis.

* * *

Communism: Enslaving people, with utopian promises of liberty *and* equality.

Liberalism: Pauperizing people, with utopian promises of prosperity.

Therapeutism: Pathologizing people, with utopian promises of health.

* * *

Catholicism, Communism, Nazism, Therapeutism, Despotism, Liberty under Law, and so forth refer to social arrangements, to systems of ordering life. None is true or false. Each is good for some people, and bad for others.

We support or oppose a particular political system or social order because we regard it as just or unjust, because we believe it confers special benefits or harms on persons who ought to be or ought not be so benefited or harmed.

The term political or social "reform" conceals the fact that the reformer's aim is to transfer benefits and harms from some people to some other people.

* * *

During the Middle Ages, when Christianity ruled the human mind, man was over-spiritualized, exemplified by the Roman Catholic prohibitions against dissecting the dead and healing the sick by other than spiritual methods. The dominant ideology proclaimed that the everlasting life of the spirit in heaven or hell was more important than the fleeting life of the body on earth, and people often behaved as if they believed it.

Today, when Medical Scientism rules the human mind, man is over-animalized, exemplified by the dogmatic belief that behavior is caused by, and can be explained in terms of, chemical and physical processes in the brain and that mental illness annuls moral responsibility. The dominant ideology proclaims that maintaining and prolonging the life of the visible and tangible body is more important than cultivating the integrity of the invisible and intangible human spirit, and people often behave as if they believe it.

Thus, there is now, as there was formerly, an imbalance between body and spirit, science and religion.

Christianity was invaluable for raising man's moral sensibility and laying the foundation for individualism and freedom; but it was worthless for advancing man's understanding and mastery of the physical universe, including his own body.

Science is invaluable for advancing man's understanding and mastery of the physical universe; but it is worthless for raising, or even maintaining, man's moral sensibility or helping him cope with ethical problems.

* * *

When an American politician running for office says "I want to serve my country," what he really means is "I want the country to be at my service."

* * *

Masses of men can feel equally poor, but not equally rich. In proportion as we raise the value of equality in politics, we lower the value of liberty and responsibility.

* * *

If Smith wants employment but cannot get it, we don't say the government is depriving him of a job he needs; however, if Smith wants medical care but cannot get it, we say the government is depriving him of the treatment he needs.

With respect to employment, we rely on the capitalist model: we eschew coercion and seek solution in voluntary contract; however, with respect to medical care, we rely on the communist model: we embrace coercion and seek solution in statism.

This choice poses a far greater threat to our liberty and "American way of life" than the military might of the Soviet Union ever did.

* * *

In 1843, the Marquis de Custine observed: "The political state of Russia may be defined in one sentence: it is a country in which the government says what it pleases, because it alone has the right to speak."[5]

In the modern totalitarian society, this remains the case: only the right man has the right to speak, and what he says is defined as the truth.

In the modern democracy, everyone has the right to speak, but the situation is not much better: when the right man utters lies, it is accepted as truth; and when the wrong man tells the truth, it is dismissed as a lie.

* * *

During election campaigns, the American people and press talk about nothing but how politicians lie and deceive the public. Once installed in office, both the people and the press treat politicians as if they were incapable of uttering a falsehood.

Ironically, the opposite generalization is closer to the mark. While campaigning, politicians tell us at least some truths—about their opponents. Once elected, however, no politician has any interest, as long as he is in office, in uttering another honest word.

* * *

In the classic tale about the emperor's finely woven clothes, a child reveals that the emperor is unclothed. That makes him a naked emperor. The point of the story, of course, is not only that the emperor is naked, but also that he is a liar.

* * *

People dream of making the virtuous man powerful, so they can depend on him. Since they cannot do that, they pretend that the powerful man is virtuous and glory in being victimized by him.

After the secular savior—Robespierre, Hitler, Stalin—is safely in his grave, the people glory once more in denouncing him as a betrayer of their trust.

Then the people repeat the cycle.

* * *

Jewish and Muslim polity begin with the faithful surrendering their freedom to God, through the covenant between God and Abraham. Its symbol is circumcision.

English polity begins with the nobles demanding their liberty and rights in opposition to the sovereign's total power. Its symbol is the Magna Carta.

In one vision, the ideal leader is God's agent and the people are his favorite children.

In the other, the ideal leader is *primus inter pares* (first among equals) and the people are independent adults.

It is foolish to believe that people who differ greatly in their religion and tradition nevertheless all want to live under the same sort of political system, and that that system is American-style democracy.

* * *

People can sympathize with the suffering of a persecuted individual, but not with that of a persecuted group.

The fate of a particular victim, an Alfred Dreyfus or Anne Frank, generates more interest and compassion than does the fate of millions of murdered Armenians or Jews.

There are martyred individuals, but there are no martyred groups or nations.

* * *

Most people cannot accept the human condition—the fact of man's dual nature, partly physical, partly spiritual.

Man's unwillingness to accept himself as a physical being is manifested by the denial of death and the affirmation, as a reality, of life in the hereafter. His unwillingness to accept himself as a spiritual being is manifested by the denial of human diversity and depravity and the affirmation, as a reality, of the fundamental uniformity and decency of human nature (spoiled only by demons or mental diseases).

Scientific medicine could not come into being until educated persons were willing to accept the finiteness of their physical selves: only then could they begin to study the human body as a material object.

Mutatis mutandis, ethical politics cannot come into being until educated persons accept the spiritual diversity and potential depravity of human beings: only then can we begin to try building a civilized and peaceful society, truly tolerant of personal differences and scrupulously protective of individual rights.

* * *

People fear and reject true diversity. The belief that there is only one right way to live—to regulate religious, political, sexual, medical affairs—is the root cause of the greatest threat to man: members of his own species bent on a quest for salvation, security, or sanity.

* * *

Addiction, obesity, and self-starvation are political problems: each condenses and expresses a contest—between the individual and some other person or persons in his environment—over the control of the individual's body and mind.

* * *

The traditional scapegoat was deprived of life, liberty, and property. Poor women, called witches, were put to death. Rich Jewish merchants, called Christ-killers or well-poisoners, were dispossessed and usually deprived of their liberties and lives as well.

Since the end of the Second World War, we have developed a new way of using scapegoats: instead of *taking* away their life, liberty, or property, we *give* them entitlements.

The modern American scapegoat is not persecuted—he is pampered. The goal is not to liquidate him, but to render him into an object of loathing.

Instead of eliminating the scapegoat from the body politic, he is now incorporated into it as an irreparably defective subhuman object that provides lucrative work and self-enhancing worry for a vast corps of social fixers and teachers of self-esteem, whose job is to encourage the scapegoats to esteem their disreputable selves.

* * *

Thomas Jefferson, Inaugural Address (1801): "Sometimes it is said that man cannot be trusted with the government of himself. Can he, then, be trusted with the government of others?"[6]

Obviously not.

Jefferson's warning underscores the basic contradiction between democracy and psychiatry, that is, between a polity based on the people's free choice of elected representatives, and a deterministic psychiatry based on the premise that people are incapable of free choice.

* * *

Juvenal (circa 60-130): *"Quis custodiet ipsos custodes?"* ("Who shall guard the guardians?"). History answers: no one.

This is the central problem of politics.

Power

Formerly, people victimized themselves by attributing medical powers to priests. Now, they victimize themselves by attributing magical powers to physicians.

Faced with persons endowed with such powers—and, of course, benevolence—men and women are inclined to submit themselves to them with that blind trust whose inexorable consequence is that they make slaves of themselves, and tyrants of their "protectors."

* * *

Some critics say I am hostile to medicine and physicians. They are wrong. I am hostile only to the power of the medical profession and of physicians.

Jefferson believed that doctors of divinity ought to have authority (if their parishioners deem them worthy of it), but no power. I believe that doctors of medicine ought to have authority (if their patients deem them worthy of it), but no power.

Prevention

Parental and political protections that prevent adults from failing also prevent them from succeeding. This is why parents who want dependent children and politicians who want ineffectual adults refuse to learn this lesson.

* * *

Unwanted pregnancy and unwanted lung cancer could, in principle, be prevented by prohibiting heterosexual, genital intercourse for couples who do not want to have (more) children and smoking.

Such sanctions would be far more harmful to the human condition than the problems they seek to prevent. The same is true for drug prohibition.

Property

Property is more tangible than health and, unlike health, gives the self the power to command others without coercing them. This why we ought to value the right to property more highly than the "right to health."

* * *

Skin separates the body from its physical environment; without enough of it—as in the case of a severe burn—the body perishes.

Money separates the person from his social environment; without enough of it—as in the case of utter destitution—the person perishes.

Psychiatric Anarchy

Official psychiatry regards the absence of psychiatric coercion as "psychiatric anarchy."

Malcom Lader, a distinguished British psychiatrist and author, writes: "The loudest voice urging that psychiatrists should not have the right to compulsory detention of their patients belongs to Thomas Szasz, Professor of Psychiatry at the State University of New York at Syracuse.... The key to Szasz's facile espousal of psychiatric anarchy lies in his admission that he sees patients only in an office practice: that is, people who come to him with their psychiatric problems."[7]

No medical practitioner other than a psychiatrist would be criticized by his colleagues for seeing only voluntary patients.

Lader's criticism, typical of the profession, supports my view that official psychiatry is synonymous with psychiatric slavery and illustrates iconoclast Edward Abbey's observation: "Fantastic doctrines (like Christianity or Islam or Marxism) require unanimity of belief. One dissenter casts doubt on the creed of millions. Thus the fear and the hate; thus the torture chamber, the iron stake, the gallows, the labor camp, the psychiatric ward."[8]

Psychiatric Drugs

Working Americans take Prozac to make them feel better. Nonworking Americans are forced to take Haldol to make others feel better.

* * *

Psychiatrists justify forcibly drugging mental patients as "life-saving treatment." This rationalization for psychiatric coercion led a federal appeals court to rule that state officials "can force a prisoner on death row to take antipsychotic medication to make him sane enough to execute."

The prisoner, Charles Laverne Singleton, cannot be put to death because psychiatrists declared him "psychotic," and because of "a

United States Supreme Court decision that prohibits the execution of the insane."[9]

Psychiatrist

The seriously sick medical patient is in a hospital bed. The physician caring for him at the bedside practices "clinical medicine," and is called a "clinician."

The seriously sick mental patient is not in a hospital bed; he is in the locked ward of a mental hospital. The psychiatrist incarcerating him in a *de facto* prison practices "carceral psychiatry," and ought to be called a "carcerian."

(The term "clinical" comes from the Greek "*klinikos*," for bed. The term "carceral," meaning related to the prison, is obsolete; it is listed in the *Oxford English Dictionary*, but not in *Webster's*.)

* * *

Psychiatrists talk neurology, and practice criminology.

* * *

Policemen subdue with arms, psychiatrists, with analogies.

* * *

Psychiatrist: 1. Existential scavenger masquerading as doctor; the purveyor of popular patent medicines, called "psychotropic drugs"; myrmidon of the therapeutic state. 2. Physician specializing in the diagnosis and treatment of nondiseases.

* * *

Fake doctors—psychiatrists and psychologists—say they "work with" patients.

Real doctors—cardiologists and surgeons—never use that phrase.

Why? Because real doctors *work with* their colleagues, not their patients.

* * *

Why can't psychiatrists relinquish coercion? Because they perceive coercing patients suffering from mental illness as intrinsic to their professional duties and identities, exactly as surgeons perceive cutting into the bodies of patients suffering from acute appendicitis as intrinsic to their professional duties and identities.

A surgeon who rejects operating on patients with acute appendicitis would not be considered a surgeon. Similarly, a psychiatrist who rejects incarcerating patients with severe depression against their will is not considered a psychiatrist.

This is why, although there are many branches of psychiatry—such as addiction psychiatry, child psychiatry, and forensic psychiatry—there is no branch of psychiatry called "non-coercive psychiatry."

The analogy with surgery holds: there is abdominal surgery, gynecological surgery, and neurosurgery, there is no non-surgical surgery. As surgery is cutting the body, psychiatry is coercing the person.

* * *

When a person asserts that he is Jesus, the psychiatrist does not believe that he is Jesus and does not refer to him as Jesus. He refers to him as a "mental patient" or "schizophrenic."

When a mental patient asserts that he "hears voices," the psychiatrist believes that the patient hears voices and refers to him as a "voice-hearer."

Both of these claims are patently false. The patient is not Jesus and he does not hear voices. He articulates these strategic, self-deceiving falsifications—in one case, of his identity, in the other, of his talking to himself—to enhance his importance and self-esteem.

* * *

Psychiatrists are in the business of legitimizing and delegitimizing claims, such as "I have been abducted by aliens" or "the FBI is out to get me."

They do this, however, not by marshaling evidence for or against the validity of the claim, as we do when, for example, someone says that the Eiffel Tower is in Berlin; instead, they do it by *examining the mind of the claimant and then making a "diagnosis" that cannot be refuted.*

* * *

The psychiatrist is a physician who uses the power of the state to deprive innocent individuals of liberty, in their own best interest.

The antipsychiatrist is a physician who would like to use the power of the state to limit psychiatrists and patients to engage only in those consensual psychiatric relations of which they approve.

Terms such as "libertarian psychiatrist" and "libertarian antipsychiatrist" are oxymorons.

Psychiatry

Psychiatry may be public and coercive or private and contractual. The task of the public psychiatrist stands in the same relation to the task of the private psychiatrist as the task of the district attorney stands to the task of the defense attorney.

As long as people speak of "psychiatry" as if it were a single, homogeneous medical specialty, similar to dermatology or ophthalmology; as long as both law and medicine refuse to separate public-coercive psychiatry from private-contractual psychiatry—there can be no meaningful debate about mental illness or mental health policy.

* * *

Psychiatry rests on the abolition of the distinction between public health and private health—that is, between protecting society from disease and disease-causing agents, and protecting the individual from disease, with the individual's consent.

* * *

Equating voluntary with involuntary psychiatry, contractual with coercive psychiatry is like equating ally and adversary, freedom and slavery, sex between consenting adults and rape, philanthropy and theft, suicide and murder.

* * *

Anglo-American law assumes, as a matter of fact, that the relationship between a person and a legal agent of the state is adversarial. The student of law is taught the duties and roles of both prosecuting attorney and defense attorney. Both jobs are legitimate and proper.

Anglo-American psychiatry assumes, as a matter of law and psychiatry, that the relationship between a person and a psychiatric agent of the state is therapeutic. The student of psychiatry is taught only the duties and roles of psychiatrist administering treatment; the psychiatrist has no other legitimate duties or roles. Only the job of the coercive psychiatrist is legitimate and proper. The psychiatrist who tries to help the coerced "patient" reject the patient role is likely to be cast out of the profession as a "renegade" and rejected by the court as an expert.

All the so-called ethical problems of psychiatry flow from this source.

* * *

In physics, we use the same laws to explain why airplanes fly, and why they crash.

In psychiatry, we use one set of laws to explain sane behavior, which we attribute to reasons (choices), and another set of laws to explain insane behavior, which we attribute to causes (diseases).

To overcome this impasse, reductionists insist on explaining all behavior by reference to causes, that is, brain function, while existentialists (as I interpret the term) endeavor to explain all behavior by reference to reasons, that is, choices.

* * *

Carl von Clausewitz (1780-1831), the Prussian military philosopher, defined war as "the continuation of diplomacy by other means."

Psychiatry is the continuation of politics by other means: It is the control and care of society's unwanted by means of drugs, housing, and the other pseudotherapeutic methods of the mental health professions.

* * *

The distinction between contractual and institutional psychiatry is in the process of being eroded.

The psychiatrist's role as agent of social control is incompatible with his role as agent of the patient.

Voluntary psychiatry is becoming an anachronism.

Involuntary psychiatry—increasingly disguised as, and confused with, voluntary psychiatry—is becoming the medical-legal standard for what constitutes the only professionally proper kind of psychiatric practice.

* * *

Real doctors control diseases, not persons.
Fake doctors (psychiatrists) control persons, not diseases.

* * *

Medical drugs control/influence diseases.
Psychiatric drugs control/influence behavior.

* * *

The business of psychiatry is to provide society with excuses disguised as diagnoses, and with coercions justified as treatments.

* * *

Psychiatry offers solutions to problems of housing by camouflaging them as problems of health: it defines some of the homeless as "mentally ill," confines them in institutions called "hospitals," and justifies forcible incarceration and decarceration as "medical treatment."

* * *

Voltaire: "Superstition is to religion what astrology is to astronomy, the very foolish daughter to a very wise mother."[10]
The relationship of psychiatry to medicine is similar.

* * *

There are students who don't study, workers who don't work, but there are, today, no patients who are not sick. Patients who have no bodily illness are considered to have a mental illness.

* * *

Psychiatry is the sewer into which modern societies discharge their insoluble moral and social problems. As sewers pollute the waters into which they empty, so psychiatry, emptying into medicine, pollutes the care and cure of the sick.

* * *

Ostensibly, the agenda of psychiatry is diagnosing and treating patients suffering from mental diseases.

Actually, its agenda is treating mental patients like criminals, and criminals like mental patients, degrading both, and depriving both of liberty and responsibility.

* * *

Formerly, it was considered ethical to oppress and exploit the Other by forcibly enslaving or enserfing him.

Today, it is ethical to do so by psychiatrically ensickening him.

* * *

For centuries, mental patients, like slaves, had obligations but no rights. Now, like despots, they have rights but no obligations. This sort of "psychiatric reform" epitomizes the irresolvable conflict between the principles of a free society and the principles of psychiatry.

* * *

Deinstitutionalization is the name of the policy of forcibly relocating mental hospital patients in publicly supported domiciles not called "hospitals" but still under mental health auspices. The victims remain under the domination of their victimizers.

After World War II, we did not speak of the deinstitutionalization of Jews in German concentration camps or of Japanese in American relocation camps.

The prisoners were freed: the shackles imposed on them by their adversaries were removed and they were restored to the same legal status as their liberators.

Self-styled psychiatric protectors of mental patients must do the same for persons imprisoned in mental hospitals.

* * *

The latest "reform" in the history of psychiatry that harms the mental patient in the name of helping him is his forcible eviction from the hospital that has become his home.

Persons who want to stay out of mental hospitals continue to be incarcerated in them. At the same time, persons who want to stay in mental hospitals are now "discharged" from them against their will.

The result is that the prison function of the mental hospital has remained unchanged and its asylum function has become progressively eroded.

* * *

The doctrine of the "right to treatment," promoted by self-seeking public-interest lawyers in the 1960s, led, in the 1980s, to the denial of asylum, deceptively called "deinstitutionalization," and to the latest form of psychiatric enslavement, called "outpatient commitment."

* * *

An old psychiatric witticism: The neurotic builds castles in the air, the psychotic lives in them, and the psychiatrist collects the rent.

Addendum: The psychiatrist builds a profession and a prison system on a metaphor, the neurotic seeks solace in them, and the psychotic is sentenced to them.

* * *

As World War II ended, basking in their newfound status, psychiatrists promised to humanize medicine. Instead, they medicalized problems in living.

* * *

From the admission note in a psychiatric hospital record: "Patient has not been auditorily hallucinated."

This phrase exemplifies the transformation of a person from subject into object, from a moral agent who experiences his being in the world and reports on it into a thing on which natural events impinge, like rain falling on a rooftop.

It is precisely this transformation that permits, promotes, and perpetuates the relentless victimization of psychiatric patients by psychiatric doctors through the guise of psychiatric diagnoses and treatments.

* * *

The scapegoater accuses a person of a wrong he did not commit; the psychiatrist forgives and punishes him for it.

* * *

Insanity plea: psychiatric excuse; attributing criminal acts to mental illness.

* * *

Legal insanity: disease caused by being charged with a serious crime, usually murder, treated by means of acquittal as not guilty and indefinite imprisonment in a hospital for the criminally insane.

* * *

Psychiatric diagnosis: The psychiatrist's statement about the patient, useful for the psychiatrist.

* * *

Psychiatric expert testimony: Mendacity masquerading as medicine.

* * *

Psychiatric nosology: A dictionary of defamations disguised as diagnoses.

* * *

Psychiatric symptom: The patient's statement about himself, translated into psychiatric jargon useful for the psychiatrist.

* * *

Psychiatric training: The ritualized indoctrination of the young physician into the theory and practice of psychiatric fraud and force.

* * *

Psychiatry: Conflict without acknowledged adversaries.

* * *

Psychohistory: The vilification of despised historical figures, presented as the products of impartial psychiatric-historical research; rarely, the glorification of revered historical figures, presented the same way.

* * *

Psychopathology: Problems in living renamed as mental diseases.

* * *

Psychotherapy: The psychiatric mystification and management of problems in living renamed as treatments.

* * *

Psychosomatic medicine: The medical philosophy according to which bodily diseases are mental, and mental diseases, physical.

* * *

Psychiatry: an ostensibly medical discipline whose subject matter is lies.

Lie #1. The participants' official names: one party is called "patient," even though he is not ill, of the other is called "therapist," even though he is not treating any illness.

Lie #2. The discipline's mendacious official language: psychiatric "diagnosis," "prognosis," and "treatment."

Lie #3. The lies that, like shadows, follow ex-mental patients through the rest of their lives: the record of psychiatric convictions, called "bipolar illness," "schizophrenia," and so forth; of imprisonments, called "hospitalization."

* * *

The medical model (of psychiatry). The claim that:

- mental diseases are proven or putative brain diseases;
- mental diseases are medical problems and hence only psychiatrists ought to be allowed to treat persons suffering from such diseases;
- mental patients are dangerous to themselves and others and do not know what is in their own best interests; it is the psychiatrist's duty to forcibly restrain and treat them.

* * *

Psychiatry deals with persons, medicine with bodies. Psychiatry is unsuccessful precisely for the same reason that medicine is successful, because it takes a materialist standpoint towards its subject matter.

* * *

Political-economic conditions necessary for the practice of contractual/non-coercive psychiatry (secular cure of souls): 1. Repeal of commitment laws. 2. Separation of psychiatry and the state.

* * *

"War is the health of the state," said Randolph Bourne.[11]

War is the ultimate *raison d'être* of the state, the rhetoric of "protecting the national interest" justifying a virtually unlimited extension of the size and scope of governmental activities. The sense of national emergency engendered by war transforms the destruction of dissident opinion into patriotism.

Similarly, psychosis is the health of psychiatry.

Psychosis is the ultimate *raison d'être* of psychiatry, the rhetoric of "protecting the patient's best interests" justifying a virtually unlimited extension of the size and scope of therapeutic activities. The sense of psychiatric emergency engendered by psychosis transforms the deprivation of liberty into hospitalization and therapy.

* * *

Psychiatrists accuse me of "withholding treatment" from "severely ill mental patients who deny that they are ill."

By definition, such persons do not want to be psychiatric patients and do not want psychiatric treatments. To accuse a psychiatrist of "withholding treatment" from such persons is like accusing a priest of withholding the last rites from persons who deny they are Catholics and that they are dying.

* * *

How do psychiatrists justify the claim that the psychiatrist who does not coercively drug a patient with bipolar illness or schizophrenia—even against the patient's explicit protests—is "withholding treatment"? This is how:

"If and when we identify the infections [that cause schizophrenia], we will have much more specific treatments for these diseases," explains E. Fuller Torrey, head of the Stanley Foundation, in an interview in *American Medical News*, the American Medical Association's official newspaper:

> It could mean a dramatic change for someone like his sister, who has spent

> most of her life hospitalized, at one point for 25 straight years. Even though antipsychotic medications make a difference, she has never responded well to them.... "I can argue [says Torrey] that every time [civil libertarians] protect the civil liberties of a woman with schizophrenia who is living on the streets, [they] are devaluing her.... By getting her involuntarily treated, and successfully treated so that she is able to live a more normal life on medication, I am doing exactly the opposite."[12]

* * *

Freedom of religion means freedom to worship according to one's conscience—and freedom to deny the reality of God.

Freedom of psychiatry ought to mean freedom to seek psychiatric treatment according to one's judgment—and freedom to deny the reality of mental illness.

* * *

Religion and psychiatry are institutions and methods for regulating human behavior. Each does so by precept, example, and alliance with the coercive power of the state.

God is the key justificatory-rhetorical term in religion. Mental illness plays the same role in psychiatry.

A person may obey the rules of religion/psychiatry voluntarily or he may be compelled to obey them by the coercive apparatus of the state.

* * *

The power of both religion and psychiatry lies in validating the denial of something obvious but too painful to acknowledge.

Religion validates the denial of the finality of death, psychiatry, the denial of personal responsibility.

It is proven beyond a shadow of a doubt that Jones has deliberately killed another person: The psychiatrist declares that Jones is not guilty of the crime.

It is clear beyond a shadow of a doubt that Jones is imprisoned: The psychiatrist declares that Jones is hospitalized.

It is established, as far as medical science can establish anything, that Jones is free of any significant abnormality of the structure and function of his body: The psychiatrist declares that Jones suffers from a life-threatening disease, called "dangerousness to self or others."

* * *

Religion and psychiatry rest on falsehoods or "lying truths."[13] Only science rests on truths or approximations to truths.

When an apple ripens, it falls to the ground; it does not fly up toward the sky.

When parents have a child who grows up to be a loving, successful adult, financially independent of them, they are proud of him. When they have a child who grows up to be an unloving, unsuccessful adult, financially dependent on them, they are embarrassed by him. Modern psychiatric science rests on the premise that such a perpetually dependent child-adult is "ill" and is ill in a way that makes him especially beloved by his parents. The proper way to speak of such a person is to call him "our loved one." This term is reserved for mental patients. Adult children suffering from arthritis or diabetes are not called "loved ones."

It is this lie that supports the belief that parents of "schizophrenic" children are especially knowledgeable about psychiatry and are the best spokespersons for the cause of mental health. In the media, such parents, discoursing about their "loved ones," interpret psychiatry for the public. In the Senate, such senators sponsor mental health legislation expanding legal control over mental patients and increasing spending on mental health. Senator Peter Domenici (R-N.M.) is such a senator.

In September 2002, Senator Domenici and Clare, his "schizophrenic" daughter, were the subjects of a sensitively written feature article in the *New York Times Magazine*. The excerpt below requires no comment.

> Domenici had been sitting beside me in an armchair in his Washington office, chatting about a re-election race that is causing him little anxiety. But when the conversation shifted to his family, and then specifically to his 40-year-old daughter, Clare, he rose abruptly and moved away, putting his solid senatorial desk between us.... When we talked in his office, I asked Domenici if he kept a picture of Clare in the extensive gallery of family photos behind his desk. "Sure," he said. Then he peered over the top of his glasses and rooted around. "Hmmm," he said. "Well. Hmmm. Well. I guess I don't have her here, and I'll have to fix that."[14]

* * *

In pre-Freudian psychiatry, the elephant in the room was sex. In post-Freudian psychiatry, it is power.

* * *

When Hobbes and Jefferson talked about the church, virtually everyone understood that they were talking about politics (power), not religion (morality).

Today, when politicians and psychiatrists talk about psychiatry, virtually no one understands that they are talking about politics (power), not medicine (healing).

Traditionally, Englishmen and Americans assumed that power in the hands of priests is misplaced. Today, they assume that power in the hands of psychiatrists is in the best hands.

So long as this remains true, there can be no genuine psychiatric reform.

* * *

Anti-psychiatrists and their followers are inconsistent and dishonest when they claim that there is no mental illness, but they know how to treat it; in other words, when they assert that *psychopathology* is not real/literal disease, but *psychotherapy/conversation* is a real/literal treatment for it.

Former mental patients and so-called mental patient liberation movements display an analogous inconsistency and dishonesty: they reject attributing mental illness to persons in order to deprive them of *liberty,* but eagerly accept such an attribution in order to secure monetary payment for persons disabled by the non-existing disease as well as in order to excuse criminals of *responsibility* for their lawless behavior.

* * *

Psychiatrists are in a hopeless fix. They cannot become honest professionals so long as they pretend to be physicians diagnosing and treating mental diseases. Yet they cannot acknowledge that they are advocates and adversaries in human conflicts and curers of souls in distress, lest they lose their credibility and status as medical doctors.

* * *

Psychiatric expert testimony in the courtroom: professional eminence masquerading as scientific evidence.

* * *

Psychiatry execrates self-induced chemical euphoria as "substance abuse," and exalts medically-induced chemical dysphoria as "psychiatric treatment."

* * *

Freud said that psychoanalysis helps the patient to exchange neurotic misery for ordinary unhappiness. *Mutatis mutandis*, somatic treatments help the patient to exchange ordinary unhappiness for the miseries of psychiatric cures.

* * *

Lewis L. Judd, former director of the National Institute of Mental Health: "The whole premise [of psychiatry] now is that profoundly disordered behavior is a psychobiological phenomenon. It manifests itself in behavior, but it's got to be related to dysfunctional mechanisms in the brain."[15]

This is a restatement, in contemporary language, of the belief of alienists that mental illnesses are brain diseases.

All behavior "must be related to the brain." Accordingly, asserting that disordered behavior is related to *dysfunctional* brain mechanisms implies that behavior considered not disordered behavior is related to *functional* brain mechanisms.

However, this cannot be true because the human brain is essentially the same in different cultures and at different times, but what counts as "profoundly disordered behavior" varies from culture to culture and from time to time. Only a few years ago, homosexuality was considered a severe mental illness in the United States.

* * *

If the psychiatric claim that mental diseases are brain diseases were true, we would, in fact, have two branches of neurology—two distinct medical specialties dealing with brain diseases: one type of neurologist, called "neurologist," to deal with brain diseases as brain diseases; and another type, called "psychiatrist," to deal with brain diseases as mental diseases.

No other medical specialty is similarly duplicated. We do not have one gynecology for housewives, and another for prostitutes; one pharmacology for law-abiding persons, another for criminals.

We have seemingly two classes of brain disease specialists because neurologists have patients, whereas psychiatrists have prisoners. Neurologists help their patients control *their* diseases, for example, epilepsy. Psychiatrists help families and the police control *troublesome persons*, denominated as "patients," for example, dangerous schizophrenics.

* * *

Psychiatry is the homeopathy of the mind-brain. Both systems claim to be based on science; both are often effective in treating non-existing diseases.

Ambrose Bierce: "Homeopathy, n. A school of medicine midway between Allopathy and Christian Science. To the last, both the others are distinctly inferior, for Christian Science will cure imaginary diseases and they can not."[16]

* * *

"Surviving spouses' depression studied," announces a typical headline celebrating the glories of psychiatric research.[17]

We are not likely to see a headline announcing, "Surviving spouses' elation studied."

* * *

The psychotic lacks personal self-esteem. For good reasons, he cannot admire himself as a person and must, therefore, fabricate imaginary grounds for self-esteem or perish.

The psychiatrist lacks professional self-esteem. For good reasons, he cannot admire himself and must, therefore, fabricate imaginary grounds for self-esteem or perish.

Thus do psychotic and psychiatrist fabricate their insane delusions and their medical theories of insanity, each as fantastic as the other, each as impervious to refutation by logical reasoning or empirical evidence as the other.

* * *

With increasing zeal, psychiatrists insist that mental diseases are brain diseases. They do not seem to realize that the logical consequences of this claim are as inimical to the identity of psychiatry as a distinct profession as are the consequences of my claim that mental illness is a myth. Here is why.

Neurology is the medical specialty devoted to the study, diagnosis, and treatment of diseases of the nervous system—brain, spinal cord, peripheral nerves.

Psychiatry is the medical specialty devoted to the study, diagnosis, and treatment of diseases of the mind—schizophrenia, depression, substance abuse.

If mental diseases are brain diseases, then psychiatry would/should be a part of neurology. If scientific and judicial authorities would recognize this to be true, medical schools would/should teach neurology, but not psychiatry; courts would/should recognize neurology, but not psychiatry; and the government and insurance companies would/should pay for the treatment of neurological illnesses, but not for the treatment of mental illnesses.

* * *

Kenneth Minogue: "Ideology is a form of theoretical conscription: *everyone*, by virtue of class, sex, race or nation, is smartly uniformed and assigned to one side or the other."[18]

Minogue's fine characterization of ideology—although it omits mental illness as one of the most important contemporary criteria for classifying persons—supports my contention that psychiatry is an ideology.

* * *

In a free society, an adult may be coerced only for the benefit of society—by the police, if he is suspected of a crime, and by the judge, if he is convicted of one. He is not supposed to be coerced for his own benefit—by educational authorities, to learn; by religious authorities, to be pious; or by medical authorities, to be treated for bodily illness. Yet, he is coerced by psychiatric authorities, to be treated for mental illness.

* * *

A psychiatrist's diagnosis of a person as "mentally ill and dangerous to himself or others" ought not to be a legally legitimate ground for depriving him of liberty. I reject the principle that society has the duty to protect such a person, called "dangerous mental patient," from himself and society from the "patient"; and the practice based on and implementing it, psychiatric preventive detention called "civil commitment."

Minors, considered incompetent to manage their lives, do not have a right to vote. Adults, considered incompetent to manage their lives, ought to be similarly denied the right to manage the body politic.

In short, the term "mental illness" ought not to be treated as a synonym for "mental incompetence"; the legal control of mental illness ought to be abolished; and proceedings for incompetence ought to be treated as matters of law, not psychiatry.

* * *

Persons who want to make one or another psychiatric practice illegal are even more dangerous enemies of individual liberty and responsibility than the psychiatrists they oppose. The prohibition of a particular procedure, like the prohibition of a drug, limits the choice of every member of society and undermines the fundamental concept of the individual as a competent adult who can manage his life without the meddling of a therapeutic state.

The demand to ban, say, electroshock treatment, is similar to the demand to ban the consumption of cigarettes or marijuana.

I distinguish between objecting to psychiatric procedures because they are *coerced*, and objecting to them because they are *psychiatric*.

My objections are strictly limited to the former.

* * *

My psychiatric critics accuse me of wanting to destroy psychiatry. That is not true.

My critics proclaim that mental illness is like any other illness, hence, that psychiatry is a medical specialty like any other.

Ironically, what I want is to create a psychiatry that resembles other medical specialties, such as ophthalmology.

The ophthalmologist cannot do, and is not interested in doing, anything to the patient that the patient doesn't want done to him.

I would like to see a psychiatry in which the psychiatrist could not do, and would not be interested in doing, anything to the patient that the patient doesn't want done to him.

Psychoanalysis

Psychoanalysis:

1. The trade name of a certain kind of conversation.

2. The name of a body of speculations about life and human relations put forward by the originator of the trade name.

3. The only medical specialty in which one must be a patient before one can become a therapist.

* * *

Psychoanalytic theory: "Analytic" revelation as explanation of human behavior; rhetoric with intellectual pretensions.

* * *

Psychoanalytic treatment: Sigmund Freud: "[T]alking people into and out of things—which is what my occupation consists in."[19]

* * *

Psychoanalytic practice: Anna Freud: "[J]ust let all the millionairesses stay crazy, they don't have anything else to do."[20]

* * *

Psychoanalytic institute: A school where the faculty, composed of middle-aged and old men and women, systemically degrades and infantilizes middle-aged students who eagerly submit to this degradation ceremony in the expectation, often unfulfilled, that, after being deprived of all independent judgment and the capacity to form such judgment, they will be able to inflict a similar treatment on others, call it psychoanalysis, and charge high fees for it.

* * *

Psychoanalytic meeting: The Yom Kippur service of the secularized, scientistic faithful: instead of regaling God in Hebrew with accounts of their spiritual sinfulness, the worshipers regale each other, in the jargon of psychoanalysis, with accounts of the mental sickness of their patients.

* * *

Psychoanalytic therapy: the analyst is the coach, the patient the boxer who must get in the ring and do the fighting.

* * *

Freud on Freud: "I am actually not at all a man of science, not an observer, not an experimenter, not a thinker. I am by temperament nothing but a conquistador—an adventurer."[21]

* * *

Freud converted speech into a specimen, to be "analyzed." Dreams thus become dung, the excrement of the "mental apparatus" in which the analyst as laboratory technician searches for the pathological contents of the patient's "unconscious mind."

* * *

Moses received the laws of God from Jehovah, to whom he claimed to have had special access.

Freud received the laws of Psychology from the Unconscious, to which he claimed to have special access.

Psychoanalysis is a religion disguised as a science.

* * *

Freud made no discoveries. His achievement lay in his ability to make people view personal unhappiness as a quasi-medical problem, and conversation as a medical treatment: "The moment a man questions the meaning and value of life, he is sick...by asking this question one is merely admitting to a store of unsatisfied libido to which something else must have happened, a kind of fermentation leading to sadness and depression."[22]

Because life is choice and choice is morality, Freud's assertion illustrates his effort to medicalize all of life.

* * *

The Church and Freud displayed the same phobic, anti-erotic attitude toward sex. One saw it as temptation and weakness, leading to sin. The other, as masturbation or venereal disease, leading to sickness. The only acceptable option was "paying" for sex by marrying and having (unwanted) babies.

* * *

Freud preached strict adherence to analytic rules that he regularly violated. This sort of hypocrisy—reminiscent of the behavior of Renaissance popes, preaching celibacy by day and sleeping with concubines at night—may well be a requirement for becoming a religious leader, but ill becomes an ethical person who respects others, especially those who seek his help.

A decent psychoanalyst/psychotherapist should set rules only for himself and his patient, to which he should adhere and that he must enforce.

If other therapists want to emulate his behavior, that is their affair, not his. How others practice psychotherapy is none of his business (except as an observer of, and commentator on, the human condition).

* * *

Free association: The term the psychoanalyst uses to register his approval of the patient who talks about what the analyst wants him to talk about.

Resistance: The term the psychoanalyst uses to register his disapproval of the patient who talks about what he himself wants to talk about; also, the patient's reluctance to pay the analyst for a service the patient no longer finds useful.

* * *

Training analysis: A job interview of indefinite duration, but always lasting several years.

* * *

Training analyst: Optician fitting his patient with distorting lenses.

* * *

"The unconscious": Turf of the psychoanalytic Mafia.

* * *

Psychoanalytic treatment stands in the same relation to ordinary conversation as the Eucharist wafer stands in the relation to a cracker.

The fact that the Host is dough is overshadowed, in the mind of the faithful, by the awe and respect he feels for the Church.

The fact that psychoanalysis is dialogue is overshadowed, in the mind of the faithful, by the awe and respect he feels for Therapy.

* * *

The psychoanalyst deals with serious moral problems but lacks moral seriousness.

* * *

The satirist deflates personal pomposities by ridiculing them: he mocks folly, but respects it; he laughs, lest he weep.

The psychoanalyst inflates personal problems by solemnizing them; he diagnoses folly and debases it; he weeps, lest he laugh.

* * *

Beware of the psychoanalyst who analyzes jokes rather than laughs at them.

* * *

Confession is to free association as absolution is to interpretation, as holy water is to cigar smoke, as original sin is to the Oedipus complex, as the soul is to the mental apparatus, as the priest is to the psychoanalyst, as Jesus is to Freud.

* * *

The priest puts the penitent on his knees; the psychoanalyst puts the patient on his back.

The priest humbles the penitent, the analyst makes the patient helpless.

* * *

Aided and abetted by corrupt analysts, patients who have nothing better to do with their lives often use the psychoanalytic situation to transform insignificant childhood hurts into private shrines at which they worship unceasingly the enormity of the offenses committed against them. This solution is immensely flattering to the patients—as are all forms of unmerited self-aggrandizement; it is immensely profitable for the analysts—as are all forms pandering to people's vanity; and it is often immensely unpleasant for nearly everyone else in the patient's life.

* * *

Psychoanalysis is an attempt to examine a person's self-justifications. Hence, it can be undertaken only with the patient's cooperation and can succeed only if the patient has something to gain by abandoning or modifying his system of self-justifications.

* * *

The analyst should be a catalyst, facilitating the patient's communication and confrontation with himself: he should mediate between the patient's acknowledged and unacknowledged desires and decisions.

The analyst does not change the patient, but helps the patient to change himself.

This is one of the reasons why an outsider to the psychoanalytic situation can never know why a patient has not changed as a result of analysis: the analyst might have failed to give the patient the proper kind of help, or the patient might have preferred to remain as he was.

* * *

It is instructive to compare the differences between the roles of the psychiatrist and the psychoanalyst in Freud's Vienna with the differences between the roles, in a medieval Christian state, of a priest and a rabbi.

The psychiatrist had power: his job was to coerce psychotics to abandon their delusions, as the priest's job was to coerce heretics to renounce their false religious beliefs.

In contrast, the psychoanalyst and the rabbi lacked power: their job was to engage only in voluntary relations with patients and parishioners.

I maintain that the single most fundamental characteristic of the psychoanalyst is his principled rejection to coerce his client, or indeed engage in any action for or against him outside the boundaries of their formal meetings.

* * *

Psychoanalysis stands in the same relation to psychiatry as dialogue stands to detention, conversation to incarceration.

* * *

I believe in the value of psychoanalysis as a secular-moral "cure of souls," that is, as a wholly voluntary and reliably confidential human service, initiated and largely controlled by the client who pays for it.

Freud himself compared the psychoanalytic relationship with the Catholic confessional. If psychoanalysis is to have a future—which, in our pharmacratic culture seems doubtful—it lies in adopting that model to the needs of modern secular man, increasingly isolated from his fellow man and community, and betrayed by the therapeutic state in which he mistakenly seeks protection from the vicissitudes of life.

* * *

Psychoanalysis has nothing whatsoever to do with illness or health, medicine or treatment, or any other idea that places "professional" listening and talking within the purview of the state's licensing authority.

Psychoanalysis is a moral enterprise. The term "psychoanalytic treatment" ought to refer to a particular kind of strictly confidential, private human relationship, a type of secular "cure of souls" similar to the Catholic confessional. The analyst's duty is to listen, speak, and fulfill his contract with the client, especially in keeping the client's communications inviolably confidential and punctually collecting the fees due for his services.

Few, if any, contemporary psychoanalysts share these views. Most analysts equate psychoanalysis with psychotherapy, consider psychotherapy to be a part of psychiatry, and believe that problems in living are diseases and that verbal and nonverbal communications are treatments.

Psychology

There is no psychology. There is only biography and autobiography.

* * *

Clinical psychology: The imposture of the medical role squared.

The psychiatrist pretends to be a real doctor, diagnosing and treating real diseases. The clinical psychologist pretends to be a psychiatrist.

Not surprisingly, the public is confused about the differences between psychiatrists and clinical psychologists.

* * *

Projective test: Tealeaf reading, with pictures or stories substituted for tealeaves. Used by psychologists to prove that they are normal and their clients are crazy.

Psychopharmacology

Psychopharmacological treatment of mental illness: A physician prescribing drugs about which he knows nothing, to a patient about whom he knows even less.

* * *

In the absence of free market competition between legal and illegal psychoactive drugs—say, lithium and opium—the benefits of psychiatric drugs, as the patient defines benefit, will remain unknown and unknowable.

* * *

We call the chemicals psychiatrists prescribe for the treatment of so-called severe mental illness "antipsychotic drugs." However, since they help psychiatrists, not mental patients, we ought to call them "propsychiatric drugs."

* * *

A report in the *Village Voice*, titled "New science raises the specter of a world without regret: The guilt-free soldier," warns about the latest breakthrough in psychopharmacology, a pill that dissolves the moral sense: "Every value he learned as a boy tells him to back down, to return to base and find another way of routing the enemy. Or, he reasons, he could complete the task and rush back to start popping pills that can, over the course of two weeks, immunize him against a lifetime of crushing remorse."[23]

This piece of pharmacomythology, characteristic of our age, is extraordinarily naive. Drugs act on the body, not our moral sense.

Scientists will never develop a drug that will annul our moral sense. Nor need they do so. Such a drug was discovered thousands of years ago and has been successfully used by people everywhere: it is called "religion." Clergymen confidently assure combatants on all sides—Israelis and Palestinians, Americans and Iraqis—that God is on their side. This has successfully tranquilized billions throughout history and there is no evidence that the power of this "drug" is waning. To the contrary, it is becoming more powerful before our very eyes. (See also *Drug*)

Psychotherapy

Psychotherapy is a myth.

Psychotherapeutic interventions are metaphorical treatments that stand in the same relation to medical treatments as editing television programs stands to repairing television sets.

* * *

Psychotherapy is not something the therapist *has*, like a drug, that he *gives* the patient.

Psychotherapy is something the therapist *does:* he engages in some type of conversation with the client.

* * *

Architects design houses, not homes; homes are what people create, or fail to create, out of their houses.

Psychotherapists provide conversations, not cures; cures (of souls, now called psychotherapies or talk therapies) are what clients who engage in such conversations create, or fail to create, out of their contacts with psychotherapists.

* * *

The psychotherapist who calls his conversations with clients "patient interviews" and tape records them is like the traveler who calls foreign locales "tourist attractions" and photographs them.

Each places a gadget, a technological barrier, between himself and his experience, attenuating or extinguishing it, while at the same time telling himself that he is trying to preserve it for more perfect future recall.

By objectifying and recording his experience, each destroys precisely that which ostensibly he tries to preserve.

* * *

The best known and financially most successful psychotherapists in the United States are the faith healers—the television evangelists and syndicated talk radio "therapists."

* * *

Are mental healers brain healers like neurologists and neurosurgeons? Or like faith healers, ministers (engaged in the cure of souls), and charlatans (selling the proverbial snake oil)?

Psychiatrists claim that medical psychotherapists are brain healers. A report in *Psychiatric News*, the American Psychiatric Association's official newspaper, is grandiosely titled, "Evidence is in: Psychotherapy changes the brain." Glenn Gabbard, M.D., professor of psychiatry and director, Baylor Psychiatry Clinic and editor of the *International Journal of Psycho-Analysis*, declares: "[B]ehavior therapy and drug therapy [are] affecting the same brain areas and in the same manner.... [It is important] to get scientific results that lend credibility to psychotherapy as a real treatment."[24]

Psychotherapists are not healers, in the medical sense of the term. Whether they are charlatans or not depends on what they do and claim they do.

* * *

The term "psychotherapy" denotes diverse principles and practices of ethics couched in the idiom of treatment. Each school or type of "therapy" reflects the aspirations and values of its practitioners. Classifying psychotherapies according to what the therapist expects from the patient, I suggest we distinguish three general types:

1. Compassionate therapy: the therapist expects improvement and gratitude. "I am working to get you well."

2. Command therapy: the therapist expects obedience and awe." Do what I tell you and you will be cured."

3. Contractual therapy: the therapist expects intellectual reciprocity and payment for services. "Listen to yourself, trust yourself, and I shall try to help you change your life if and as you want it changed."

* * *

Psychotherapy cannot help but be an exercise in applied ethics. One of the most important principles that must guide persons who want to elevate the Other—not merely "accept" or even diminish him—was beautifully stated by Goethe: "If I accept you as you are, I will make you worse; however, if I treat you as though you are what you are capable of becoming, I help you become that."[25]

* * *

People seeking help from psychotherapists can be divided into two groups:

1. Persons who wish to confront their problems and change their lives by changing themselves.

2. Persons who wish to avoid the inexorable consequences of their life strategies through "therapy."

* * *

Literary anticipation of the so-called medical model of mental illness and psychotherapy: Samuel Butler began to write *The Way of All Flesh* in 1872 and completed it in 1884, about the same time that Sigmund Freud began to show interest in psychotherapy, and some ten years before the publication of Breuer and Freud's *Studies on Hysteria.*[26]

> Rome has reduced the treatment of the human soul to a science, while our own Church, though so much purer in many respects, has no organized system either of diagnosis or pathology—I mean, of course, spiritual diagnosis and spiritual pathology.... [E]ither the priest is indeed a spiritual guide, as being able to show people how they ought to live better than they can find out themselves, or he is nothing at all—he has no *raison d'être*. If the priest is not as much a healer and director of men's souls as a physician is of their bodies, what is he? The history of all ages has shown that as men cannot cure the bodies of their patients if they have not been properly trained in hospitals under skilled teachers, so neither can souls be cured of their more hidden ailments without the help of men who are skilled in soul craft—or in other words, of priests....
>
> As for men curing themselves...they can no more cure their own souls than they can cure their own bodies, or manage their own law affairs. In these last two cases they see the folly of meddling with their own cases clearly enough, and go to a professional adviser as a matter of course; surely a man's soul is at once a more difficult and intricate matter to treat, and at the same time it is

> more important to him that it should be treated rightly than that either his body or his money should be so.[27]

Butler used the "medical model" as a linguistic device to explain the function of the priest as spiritual guide. Freud used it to define psychoanalysis as a literal treatment, except when it suited his political-polemical purposes to disavow this transparent literalization of a metaphor. In 1927, he wrote: "I have assumed that psychoanalysis is not a specialized branch of medicine.... The words, 'secular pastoral worker,' might well serve as a general formula for describing the function of the analyst."[28]

* * *

Why would a psychotherapist want to formulate rules for other therapists to follow? How would the successful propagation of such rules benefit him, except by aggrandizing him as a great rule-maker? But making rules for others is, *par excellence*, an enterprise in heteronomy, incompatible with valuing autonomy.

* * *

The autonomous psychotherapist's role vis-a-vis his client is like the court jester's vis-a-vis the monarch: with sympathy and tact, he confronts the client with painful reality; the client retains complete control over whether or not he wants to listen to what the therapist is telling him.

* * *

Voltaire said: "No priest should ever deprive a citizen of the least prerogative on the pretext that this citizen is a sinner, because [the priest]...should pray for sinners, and not judge them."[29]

This rule defines the role of the autonomous psychotherapist: No psychotherapist should ever deprive a citizen of the least prerogative on the pretext that this citizen is mentally ill, because the psychotherapist should listen and talk to patients, not deprive them of liberty or responsibility.

* * *

People with personal problems often behave like the proverbial drunk who looks for his house key under the streetlight, because that's where the light is, not because that's where the key is.

Should such a person consult an autonomous psychotherapist, the therapist's job is not to try to find the key, but to suggest to the patient that he light a match or borrow a flashlight from a neighbor and go look for his key where he dropped it.

* * *

Success in psychotherapy—that is, the ability to change oneself in a direction in which one wants to change—requires courage rather than insight.

* * *

For the psychiatrist, mental illness is brain disease; for the psychologist, behavioral disorder; for the social worker, family problem.

However much these mental health professionals might disagree about the nature of the problem before them, they all agree that psychotherapy is an effective *therapeutic* intervention and that their particular brand is the best.

* * *

During the 1950s, when psychoanalysis was fashionable, the title of a typical psychiatric article or lecture was: "The Psychodynamics of Depression."

Today, when psychopharmacology is fashionable, a typical title is: "The Drug Treatment of Depression."

* * *

Is there a cure for depression? In the medical sense, no. In the existential sense, yes.

When the person's depressing life situation improves—because of his own actions or for any other reason—his depression lifts or disappears.

* * *

All psychiatric/psychotherapeutic relations between consenting adults ought to be permissible. It is not the government's business whether "therapy" is good or bad, helpful or unhelpful.

At the same time, all psychiatric/psychotherapeutic relations that are coerced ought to be prohibited: the therapist's claim that the patient benefits from the therapy ought not be an acceptable justification for coercion under therapeutic auspices. (Psychiatric/psychotherapeutic relations between adults and children ought to be prohibited, exactly as sexual relations between adults and children are prohibited.)

In a free society, there can be no valid objection to psychotherapy between consenting adults; nor can there be any valid defense of the therapeutic rape of the patient by the therapist.

Punishment

Prisons, called "correctional institutions," are supposed to rehabilitate criminals.

Madhouses, called "mental hospitals," are supposed to treat mentally ill persons.

By denying that criminals are, in fact, punished and that mental hospital patients are not, in fact, receiving real medical treatment for real diseases, we undermine the legitimacy of punishing lawbreakers, and conceal the illegitimacy of imprisoning persons innocent of lawbreaking.

* * *

There is much speculation nowadays about whether lawbreakers should be punished or treated. This problem disappears if we divorce the concepts of punishment and treatment from the subject's condition at the end of the intervention.

Punishment is an intervention to which the subject, called "criminal," submits by force. Treatment is an intervention to which the subject, called "patient," submits by choice.

Punishment may result in rehabilitation and be judged helpful by the criminal and others. Treatment may result in disability or death and be judged harmful by the patient and others.

The *outcome* of punishment or treatment should not confuse us about whether the intervention was forcibly coerced or freely chosen.

* * *

There can be only two responses to deviance: control or tolerance. We must either imprison or kill deviants, or tolerate and live with them.

This is the basic reason for defining persons who deprive others of life, liberty, or property as criminals, and abolishing psychiatric slavery (involuntary psychiatry).

* * *

The current liberal-psychiatric position on the death penalty is callous hypocrisy masquerading as compassionate reverence for life, except for the life of the unborn.

Revolted by the anti-death penalty cant prominently featured in the pages of the *New York Times*, a recently released Federal prisoner writes: "[The death penalty] is much kinder than a sentence of 25 years in prison.... Many death-row inmates might well choose death in lieu of a mandatory 25-year sentence.... Witness the high rate of prison suicide or attempted suicide."[30]

Opponents of the death penalty don't really care about the lives or deaths of prisoners. If they did, they would give them what I have called "the Socrates option": a choice between a painful life in prison and a painless release from it by death, by means of appropriate drugs put at their disposal by the prison authorities.[31]

Q

Quackery

Quackery: pretending to practice medicine without a license. Psychiatry: pretending to practice medicine with a license.

R

Racism

In the lexicon of contemporary political correctness, the most persuasive way to express one's condemnation of an act or habit is by calling it a "disease." Calling racism a disease is an example.

Alvin Poussaint, a black professor of psychiatry at Harvard Medical School, declares: "My position is that *extreme racism is a serious mental illness because it represents a delusional disorder.*"[1]

"'Is racism dead?" asks famed actor James Earl Jones. His answer: "'Yeah, it's dead like Prohibition made alcohol dead.'... Jones sees it [racism] as a medical issue. 'It's an addiction,' he said. 'It makes them feel good.'"[2]

* * *

Racism as mental illness: Revenge for drapetomania and dysaesthesia Aethiopis. (Drapetomania was the mental illness that made slaves run away to freedom. Dysaesthesia Aethiopis was the mental illness that made slaves "accidentally" destroy their masters' property.[3])

Rational, Rationality

1. Mentally healthy. 2. One of the most important words—along with its opposite, "irrational"—in the vocabulary of psychiatry. 3. Irrational: A judgment masquerading as a diagnosis.

* * *

In psychiatry, being a rational person is synonymous with being a sane, mentally healthy, responsible person; being an irrational person is synonymous with being an insane, mentally ill, not responsible person; and only the rational person is considered (fully) human.

In mathematics, a rational number is an integer or the quotient of an integer divided by a non-zero integer; and an irrational number is any real number that can be expressed neither as an integer nor as a quotient of an integer divided by a non-zero integer. Both types of numbers are equally real.

* * *

Who determines who or what is rational or not rational?

De facto, each person makes this judgment about ideas, information, and people for himself.

De jure, courts, psychiatrists, and psychologists determine whether a person is rational (mentally competent) or not.

Yet, psychiatrists and psychologists regularly categorize their colleagues' views as irrational. According to the distinguished British psychologist Stuart Sutherland (1927-1998), the Rorschach diagnostic test is worthless, yet it is estimated "that six million Rorschach tests are given a year—a glaring example of irrationality among psychologists."[4]

In an obituary of Sutherland, Christopher Longuet-Higgins, a colleague at the University of Sussex, wrote: "As a psychologist he could insist that people—other people—were driven by irrational impulses rather than guided by reason; but as an Oxford philosopher he could not allow that generalisation to apply to himself.... Stuart was the despair of the doctors who failed to stop him from smoking after a succession of heart operations...."[5]

* * *

The terms "rational/irrational," like the terms "sane/insane," are subjective judgments masquerading as objective, medical, scientific, verifiable assessments or determinations.

It would be more honest if instead of calling people "irrational" and "insane," we simply said that they are wrong, ignorant, credulous, gullible, fearful, conceited, smug, self-satisfied, mistaken, or know what isn't so.

Everyone holds false beliefs about some things, and no one holds false beliefs about everything.

The person whom the psychiatrist labels as "irrational" is rational. He differs from the psychiatrist in having different opinions, premises, and values.

Every adherent to a monotheistic religion believes, *ipso facto*, that adherents to the other two monotheistic religions are "irrational."

* * *

As the idea of bodily illness entails the notions of somatic lesion or dysfunction, so the idea of mental illness entails the notions of irrationality and non-responsibility.

Reality

The strongest bond to reality is loving one's child and being responsible for him.

The second strongest is loving one's work.

Reason

1. The capacity to reflect and make choices.

2. The faculty that enables us to distinguish human beings from animals, which human beings use to deny the validity of this distinction.

Redistribution

The economic liberal redistributes money, from producers to parasites.

The psychiatric liberal redistributes responsibility, from patients to psychiatrists, from psychiatrists to drug companies, and from individuals to society.

Religion

Religions are like icebergs: a tip of love and compassion at the top, and a mass of hatred and contempt at the bottom.

* * *

Religion is praised for its power to unite people in harmonious congregation. It can do that.

However, it also deserves to be condemned, but is not condemned, for its far greater power to disunite people, setting one group against another in a struggle of mutual annihilation.

* * *

Monotheism entails religious intolerance.

* * *

Religion: Vicarious conceit, megalomania, and narcissism; a tactic for de-meaning the Other.

* * *

Persons who believe that the Torah, the New Testament, or the Koran are the words of God are called "literalists" and "fundamentalists," while those who interpret them figuratively are called "liberals" and "non-fundamentalists."[6] These are evasions.

The opposite of the literal interpretation of a text is a metaphorical interpretation of it. In scholarly discussions of religion, however, such clarity is carefully avoided. Why? Because the metaphorical interpretation of an allegedly God-given text is, in plain English, an atheistic interpretation of it. If a sacred text is God's word only in the sense that the fluctuations of the stock market "speak" to financial analysts, then they are not God's words at all. In which case we may respect them as sage advice or dismiss them as mere opinion, but cannot be expected to revere them as holy revelation.

* * *

Marx called religion an "opiate." In communist hands, religion freely professed becomes a dangerous drug that must be outlawed, while religion brutally enforced becomes Scientific Marxism, which the whole world must embrace.

Freud called religion a "neurosis." In psychiatric hands, conventional religion freely professed becomes a self-destructive illness that must be cured, while the religion of psychiatry, brutally enforced, becomes a scientific treatment to which the whole world must submit.

* * *

Two of the most important western religions today are communism and psychiatry.

Each rests on the principle that human behavior is determined by scientific laws and that the individual has no free will, and on the practice of depriving individuals of the freedom to make uncoerced choices.

* * *

We can call a man a "son of a bitch," or a "son of a gun," or a "son of God." No one interprets the first two expressions literally, but many people do so interpret the third one, and disparage those who do not.

* * *

The American Constitutional doctrine of the separation of church and state means simply that religion and government are free and independent of one another.

But freedom is a burden as well as an opportunity. In this case, the burden is that religion must manage without the support of the government, and government without the support of religion. It is not surprising, then, that the lofty principle of political secularism is under unceasing assault, mainly along two fronts: taxation and psychiatry.

The Internal Revenue Service, by granting tax exemption to churches, functions as a government agency validating some belief systems as "religions," and invalidating others as "cults."

Psychiatry considers membership in a conventional church as a manifestation of mental health, and membership in a so-called cult as a manifestation of mental illness. In this way, it functions as a government agency validating some systems of belief as religions, and invalidating others as dangers to mental health and public health.

* * *

A person in a position of authority and power—parent, priest, politician, physician—can make others dependent on him or help them become dependent on themselves.

History teaches us that the person who makes others dependent on him is worshiped and remembered, whereas the person who helps others become independent is ignored and forgotten.

Responsibility

Responsibility is not a phenomenon or trait, like eye color. Instead, it is an attribution, one person ascribing moral agency to another person and adopting towards him the appropriate social regulatory principle, rewarding him for good deeds and punishing him for bad deeds.

* * *

The twentieth century has been an age of unparalleled technological progress accompanied by an unparalleled rejection of personal responsibility.

In totalitarian and free societies alike, the formula for justifying non-responsibility has been: "I was only following orders."

In the totalitarian state, the actor is not responsible because he is "only following orders" issued by his political superiors.

In the therapeutic state, the actor is not responsible because he is "only following orders" issued by his addiction, compulsion, irresistible impulses, mental illnesses, and "voices."

* * *

We have lost the ability to appreciate the difference between holding a person responsible and blaming him. When I say that a smoker is responsible for smoking, I am not necessarily blaming him for his habit or its consequences. I am simply asserting that he is the agent of his action.

If we attribute an individual's action to a cause outside of himself—a drug, disease, mental disease, poverty, injustice—we undermine our concept of responsibility, the basis of civilization. Excusing the actor from responsibility for the destructive, undesirable consequences of his conduct is tantamount to creating scapegoats to blame instead.

* * *

When I assert that we are always responsible for our behavior, this is what I mean:

- *Scenario 1.* Jones is cashing a check at a bank. A gunman puts a gun to his head and orders him to ask the teller for money or he will shoot him. Jones obeys the order. The law recognizes a condition, called "duress," that excuses his behavior. This does not mean that Jones had no choice. It means only that society does not want to punish this type of behavior. Jones is existentially, though not morally or legally, responsible for his act.

- *Scenario 2.* A gunman breaks into Jones' home, puts a gun to his head and knife in his hand, and orders him to stab his wife. Jones refuses to obey the order.

- *Scenario 3.* Jones stabs his wife, claiming that God told him she was possessed by the devil and he must kill her. Investigation reveals that, according to Jones and his wife, they had an idyllic marriage for about a year, until Jones had a nervous breakdown. He spent a few weeks in a mental hospital, was diagnosed as suffering from paranoid schizophrenia, and was told to take antipsychotic drugs. After leaving the hospital, Jones soon stopped taking the drugs. A few weeks later he stabbed his wife. Psychiatrists testify that he is not responsible for his crime because he was unable to resist obeying the "voices" he was hearing. Jones is recommitted to the hospital and the charges against him are dropped.

In a word, psychiatry and law recognize the *metaphorical duress* of what psychiatrists call "hallucinations" or "hearing voices." I reject this view.

Psychotic patients are able to resist the orders of physicians to take prescribed drugs. They are also able to resist the orders of their "voices." There is neither empirical evidence nor moral ground to support the claim that certain mentally ill persons are not responsible for their actions. People are responsible for their actions regardless of gender, race, religion, economic status, or psychiatric diagnosis.

* * *

We call the state of man before he attains knowledge of good and evil "innocence," not "ignorance."

Which raises this question: What sort of person do we have in mind when we say he does not know right from wrong and hence ought not to be punished? Do we mean a person who:

1) *never knew right from wrong?*

2) knew right from wrong and knows it now, but who, during a particular moment in time, *forgot it*?

3) knew right from wrong but has *forgotten* it and cannot possibly recover it without ingesting psychiatric drugs?

4) knew right from wrong but has no memory of it and hence no hope of ever again knowing it?

Each answer is a disguised strategy to justify controlling the subject, for a short time, a long time, or the rest of his life.

Right (see Autonomy)

Risk

"We can't close off the mountain [the Matterhorn] to reckless amateurs.... You can't stop people if they want to throw themselves off the Golden Gate Bridge," declared Richard Andenmatten, a long-time Alpine guide, after a series of mountaineering accidents.[7]

We let people risk their lives climbing mountains, because mountain climbing is not a medical matter; but we do not let people risk their lives taking drugs, because drug taking is a medical matter.

Rule of Law

Friedrich A. Hayek stated: "Under the rule of law, government can infringe a person's protected private sphere only as punishment for breaking an announced general rule."[8] If we were to follow this principle, psychiatry as we know it would disappear.

Paraphrasing Hayek, I say: Under the rule of psychiatry, government can infringe a person's protected private sphere whenever its psychiatric agents declare a person "mentally ill and dangreous to himself or others." The rule of law is thus replaced by the rule of psychiatric discretion: judicial fact-finding, trial by jury, and a finite term of incarceration in prison are replaced by mental examination, psychiatric diagnosis, and an indefinite term of incarceration in an insane asylum.

S

Sadism

We call persons who experience sexual pleasure from inflicting pain on their partners "sexual sadists."

We ought to call persons who experience professional pleasure from inflicting pain on their partners "professional sadists," exemplified by child psychiatrists and forensic psychiatrists.

Scapegoat

Man has a natural tendency to attribute calamities to scapegoats.

In the past, women called witches and people called Jews, a.k.a. "Christ-killers," occupied that role.

Today in the United States, the users of illegal drugs and "dangerous mental patients" are the scapegoats.

* * *

In the Theological State, the government claims control over the soul of man and his life in the hereafter. Those who want to assert control over their own souls and lives in the present are persecuted as heretics.

In the Communist State, the government claims control over land, factories, and labor. Those who want to assert control over their own labor and property are persecuted as capitalists.

In the Therapeutic State, the government claims control over drugs, medical care, and the health of the citizen. Those who want to assert control over their own bodies, minds, and drug use are persecuted as lawbreakers or patients.

* * *

In the "religious model" of domination, the strong controlled the Other by declaring him a "heretic."

In the "slavery model," he controls the Other by enslaving him, and in the "medical model," by diagnosing him as "mentally ill."

Schizophrenia

If you talk to God, you are praying. If God talks to you, you have schizophrenia.

* * *

If the dead talk to you, you are a spiritualist. If God talks to you, you are a schizophrenic.

* * *

When a man says he is Jesus, he is not complaining; he is boasting.

We consider his claim a symptom of illness; he considers it a stamp of greatness.

* * *

If you believe that Jesus is the son of God, your belief is regarded as a "symptom" of your being a Christian. If you believe that you are Jesus, your belief is regarded as a symptom of schizophrenia.

Because "schizophrenia" is the name of a disease, psychiatrists look for defective genes, twisted molecules, and "chemical imbalances in the brain" as its cause. If Christianity were called a disease, would psychiatrists look for its biological causes?

We will discover the chemical cause of schizophrenia when we discover the chemical cause of Christianity. No sooner and no later.

* * *

The schizophrenic's initial dramatic misbehavior—aggressiveness, hallucinations, self-neglect—are interpreted as manifestations of a disease of the brain. The fact that fifty years later he is free of any evidence of brain disease—provided he has not been subjected to "treatments" causing brain disease—is not interpreted as evidence that his earlier misbehavior was not a manifestation of brain disease.

* * *

When a man says he is Jesus or makes some other claim that seems to us outrageous, we call him psychotic and lock him up in the madhouse. Freedom of speech is only for normal people.

* * *

Hallucination is self-conversation, a speech act protected by the Constitution as freedom of speech.

Delusion is false belief, another type of speech act protected by the Constitution as freedom of religion.

Illegal *acts* based on belief, true or false, ought to be punished by the criminal law, not the mental health law.

If a man shoots his wife—because he believes, rightly, that she is unfaithful to him—he is guilty of a crime. But if he shoots her because he believes, wrongly, that she is a witch, he is acquitted as not guilty by reason of insanity, and incarcerated in a mental hospital.

In both cases, the man should be punished as a murderer. In each case, he can protect himself legally and without violence by leaving or divorcing his wife.

* * *

The psychiatrist is unable to understand what the patient says (perhaps because the patient speaks a foreign tongue). Diagnosis: schizophrenia.

* * *

We say that the schizophrenic is "mentally disturbed." The truth is that he disturbs others.

* * *

Schizophrenia is the joker in the deck of the justificatory rhetoric of psychiatry as social control. The "diagnosis" trumps all arguments and objections against imposing ostensibly therapeutic interventions on the denominated patient.

* * *

If a person's circulation fails, he has ischemia. If his kidneys fail, he has uremia. If his life fails, he has schizophrenia.

To cure ischemia, doctors transplant blood vessels. To cure uremia, they transplant kidneys. What should they transplant to cure schizophrenia?

If our life were an organ, it might be possible for doctors to repair its malfunctioning, perhaps by replacing it with another. But our life is not a part of us, it *is* us. That is why no one else can fix it when it malfunctions, or replace it when it fails.

* * *

Schizophrenia: 1. The cancer of conceit. 2. Early retirement from life. 3. Unwillingness to cooperate and be of any use to anyone. 4. Prevention of schizophrenia: modesty and self-discipline.

* * *

Schizophrenia—"the cancer of conceit": A case report from the *Journal of the American Medical Association*:

> Dr. Reynolds: Mr X is a 23-year-old man with a 5-year history of schizophrenia.... Mr X began to have social withdrawal and isolation around age 16, when he dropped out of school sports, went from being an excellent student to barely passing, and began spending much of his free time alone watching videos. He was using alcohol, cannabis, and LSD (lysergic acid diethylamide). He had progressively paranoid delusions: he believed that the Mafia was going to make him a movie star, that bystanders stared at him because they knew he was famous, and that the Mafia was broadcasting to him and controlling his mind....
>
> Mr. X. His view: ...I started getting messages from the loudspeaker in class, and I started reading between the lines and thinking when someone was talking to me that they were meaning something else, but I would actually hear that in my head.... I started thinking there was a whole conspiracy around me, thinking people were watching me, the Mafia was behind me, the Mafia was going to make me a movie star. *When you actually believe that, sometimes it's fun. You're driving around really thinking you're this next movie star. When someone looks at you, you think, "Wow, they look at me, they know who I am. I'm famous." You start enjoying it, and then it goes away and you're down there again. It's like a roller coaster ride*.... It was a big shock. When you think all that stuff is true, and all of a sudden you come back down to reality and you realize it was all in your head, it's a blow—like someone literally hit you.... I heard from asking questions and asking doctors that there's a chance if you go off the medication you might not need it. I wanted to take that chance, so I took myself off the medication. But I made a real bad mistake and I decided to substitute illegal drugs. Cocaine and ecstasy were the ones that I chose. The ecstasy calmed me down. It made me in touch with my feelings, and I could talk to anybody; anybody could talk to me....[1]

* * *

Schizophrenia—"the cancer of conceit": The case of celebrity-schizophrenic Nobel Prize winner John Nash:

> "Madness can be an escape," explains Nash in a Public Broadcasting System interview. "If things are not so good, you maybe want to imagine something better. In madness, I thought I was the most important person in the world.... To some extent, sanity is a form of conformity. And to some extent, people who are insane are non-conformists and society and their family wish that they would live what appear to be useful lives."[2]

Nash became "sick" when he decided to, and recovered when he decided he had had enough.

* * *

Schizophrenia is a non-disease, which it is impossible to cure, but from which it is easy to recover.

* * *

An editorial in the *Wall Street Journal* declares: "Refusing to recognize the reality of schizophrenia is a scandal."[3]

In the therapeutic state, indeed it is. Just as refusing to recognize the reality of the deity of Yahweh, Jesus, and Allah is a scandal in, respectively, yeshivas, Catholic schools, and madrasas.

* * *

Jones is an extra on the stage of life. He wants to be a star. He cannot become a star by making a fortune on the stock market or winning a Nobel Prize. Instead, he claims that the FBI or the Communists are watching his every move, tapping his phone, sending him coded messages. They would not be doing this if he were not a very important person.

A paranoid delusion is a problem to the so-called patient's family and friends. For the "patient," it is a solution for the problem of the meaning(lessness) of his life.

* * *

Schizophrenia: 1. Flunking life. 2. Vacation from life. 3. Strategy for being the most useless, yet most important, member of the family.

* * *

The irony of schizophrenia: The schizophrenic *thinks* he is all-powerful. Eventually, he runs afoul of the psychiatrist who *is* all-powerful over him.

* * *

Schizophrenia: hyperesthesia of the soul.
Biological treatment for schizophrenia: anesthetizing the soul.

* * *

Schizophrenia is a declaration, not a disease.

The subject asserts a conceited capitulation: "I will not exert myself for the rewards the world has to offer; I refuse to lower myself and get down into the dirt of everyday life; I am too good for that."

The psychiatrist asserts a conceited claim: "The patient is incurably ill and dangerous to himself and others; only psychiatrists are professionally qualified to deal with this, the most severe of all mental illnesses, and only they are qualified to make decisions serving the patient's best interests.

* * *

Upset by her teenage daughter's rebelliousness, a New York mother commits her to Columbia University's Psychiatric Institute (P.I.). In her memoir, the "patient" writes: "On my application for admission to P.I., asked to specify the reason for hospitalization, my mother had written: 'Rebellious behavior.' All my friends at P.I. were then diagnosed as schizophrenic.... I was never schizophrenic. Not then, not now. How could they possibly have interpreted my rage and confusion as schizophrenia?"[4]

The answer is called "standard of care." Had one of the psychiatrists assigned to treat this young woman asserted that she did not "have schizophrenia" and set her free, and had she then killed herself (or injured her mother), the psychiatrist would have faced an unwinnable malpractice suit.

* * *

In 1911, when Eugen Bleuler invented schizophrenia, the disease was said to be incurable. Since then, it has allegedly been cured with insulin coma, metrazol shock, electric shock, lobotomy, and neuroleptic drugs.

In 1988, a new cure for it was announced: the transplantation of embryonic brain tissue into the brain of the schizophrenic patient.[5]

The emperor called "schizophrenia" has, as I have remarked elsewhere, so many beautiful robes that it is unthinkable that he should not exist.[6]

* * *

The etiology of a bodily disease has to be discovered only once. After the causes of malaria, paresis, and puerperal fever were firmly established, the etiology of each became a part of its definition.

The etiology of a mental disease has to be discovered over and over again. Each time the discovery and the discoverer is celebrated; and when the discovery proves to be erroneous, the mistake is quickly forgotten.

In 1949, Egas Moniz was awarded the Nobel Prize for discovering that schizophrenia is due to reverberating electrical circuits in the frontal lobes.

Since then, psychiatrists and neuroscientists have been hailed and honored for discovering that "it" was due to genetic defects, chemical abnormalities in the brain, and lesions in the amygdala and other brain regions.

Nonexistent diseases have many causes.

* * *

Psychiatrists call schizophrenia a "thought disturbance."

By the same token, we could call heresy a "belief disturbance."

In each case, the question is: Who is disturbed—the patient/heretic, or his judges?

If the subject himself were disturbed, he would seek relief for his disturbance. He does not do that. I conclude that he is not disturbed.

If others were disturbed, they would seek relief for their disturbance. That is precisely what they do. I conclude that schizophrenia is a type of disturbing behavior that may not, but often does, constitute grounds for arrest and prosecution for crime.

My aim with respect to the political and social situation of "schizophrenics"—and mental patients generally—has been to extend to them the same protections from psychiatric coercions that "heretics" are guaranteed with respect to religious coercions.

"The real object of the [First] amendment," declared Justice Joseph Story, "was not to countenance, much less advance, Mahometanism, or Judaism, or infidelity...but to exclude all rivalry among Christian sects.... It thus cuts off the means of religious persecution (the vice and pest of former ages) and of the subversion of the rights of conscience in matters of religion."[7]

My object in urging that we extend the protections of the First Amendment to beliefs now categorized as psychiatric is not to countenance, much less advance, "crazy" beliefs, but to exclude all rivalry, with respect to what constitutes rationality, among religious, psychiatric, and other systems of beliefs. This would cut off the means of psychiatric persecution (the vice and pest of the Age of Reason) and of the subversion of the rights of conscience in matters of psychiatry.

* * *

The lover and the schizophrenic display opposite dispositions.

The lover is attached, intimate, passionate, and longs—for the Other.

The schizophrenic is detached, lonely, aloof, and is uninterested—in the Other.

These characterizations are consistent with the fact that "everyone loves a lover," whom we consider especially fortunate and lovable; and that "everyone hates a schizophrenic," whom we consider especially unfortunate and loathsome.

* * *

The person who displays the symptoms of schizophrenia often pretends that he is not an agent. He acts as if he were an object.

The psychiatrist who diagnoses a person as schizophrenic also pretends that the patient is not an agent. He treats him as if he were an object.

* * *

The so-called schizophrenic is often a person who refuses to admit that he has lived badly, is useless, guilty, or sinful. He rids himself of his bad conscience by projecting it, hence the accusing voices he hears.

Only the truth, as Jesus admonished, can set him free.

The problem—for him as well as us—is that often he does not want to be set free, because he prefers that others take care of him as a psychiatric invalid.

The more clearly we understand schizophrenia in moral terms, the more absurd it is to speak of treating persons so diagnosed as if they were sick.

* * *

Typhoid fever is an infectious, febrile disease caused by the typhoid bacillus.

Spring fever is not an illness, does not cause fever, and has no medically meaningful cause. *Webster's* defines it as: "Humorous. The lazy listless feeling that comes to persons with the first warm days of spring."

Perhaps some day dictionaries will define schizophrenia as follows: "Obsolete. A term formerly used to disguise the medical misinterpretation of the lazy, listless feeling, especially of adolescents and young adults, that comes over them with the first realization that they must stand on their own feet."

* * *

Different observers may *call* the same person a religious fanatic, a victim of political persecution, or a paranoid schizophrenic.

Each of these classifications rests on a mixture of description and judgment, much the same way as does *calling* the same glass half-full or half-empty.

If we want to assemble an adequate sample of, say, eight-ounce glasses containing four ounces of liquid, we must do so by ascertaining that the volume of liquid in each is exactly one-half its total capacity, not by what people call them. Thus, we cannot study schizophrenia biologically unless we assemble a sample of "schizophrenics" according to some objective criterion. But there is no such criterion.

Instead, psychiatrists establish who counts as a schizophrenic on the basis of the decision of "consensus groups" of experts. "Saint-makers" use the same method to establish who counts as a saint.[8]

* * *

According to psychiatric doctrine, the typical schizophrenic patient begins to manifest symptoms of his "brain disease" during late adolescence. Nevertheless, often he lives to a ripe old age in robust health, without evidence of neurological or psychological deterioration even in his seventies or eighties. This would be a truly remarkable life history for a brain disease.

The natural history of schizophrenia has engendered skepticism toward it in some psychiatrists, but not many. Few share the sentiments ably articulated by Myre Sim:

> For most of this century, on the basis of the most authoritative laboratory evidence of the time, schizophrenia has been variously attributed to degeneration of the interstitial cells of the testes, degeneration of the liver, and malfunctions of the kidneys, adrenals, and thyroid. The frontal lobes have also been implicated as have vitamin deficiencies and a variety of metabolic disorders. Yet, schizophrenics had the longest expectations of life among residents of mental hospitals and they enjoyed such rude health that they constituted the greatest security risk. You may be excused if you have concluded that all this laboratory work was done by second or third raters. Far from it. The man who provided proof of the testicular degeneration theory was elected a Fellow of the Royal Society of London and was later knighted."[9]

* * *

Psychiatrists now assert, as a certainty, that schizophrenia is a brain disease. Let us assume that "it" is. (The scare quotes are intended to alert the reader to the problematic character of what "it" is.)

In what way would that help us cope with the problems we attribute to schizophrenia or, more precisely, to schizophrenics? The truth is, it would help us only to see more clearly that the belief that schizophrenia is a brain disease conceals moral and social problems not susceptible to solution by medical research or treatment.

Suppose that a young adult diagnosed as suffering from schizophrenia refuses to study or work, neglects his health and hygiene, and perhaps even speaks about killing himself or members of his family. Would his parents, psychiatrists, and judges be justified in incarcerating him in a mental hospital against his will? Or suppose that he kills his mother, "because" he suffers from schizophrenia. Would that justify excusing his criminal behavior and incarcerating him in a mental hospital against his will?

At present, there is no biologically identifiable brain disease whose sufferers are treated in this manner by the legal system. Nor is there a brain disease whose sufferers exhibit such behaviors.

I believe that the identification of a brain disorder "responsible" for schizophrenia would compel us treat the sufferer from it the same way we treat others suffering from brain diseases. Either, they would be declared legally incompetent, like patients with Alzheimer's dementia, and cared for as we care for infants. Or they would be regarded as responsible and respectable moral agents, like patients with epilepsy, and treated legally and socially the same way as we treat diabetics and healthy persons, deserving of human rights if they obey the law, and of appropriate punishment if they do not.

* * *

In the United States today, a person has the right to refuse to give blood for an AIDS test. In short, he can prevent others from diagnosing him as having AIDS.

As matters now stand, there is no objective, biological test for schizophrenia. This makes it impossible for a person to prevent others from diagnosing him as having schizophrenia.

Suppose that the dreams of biological psychiatrists were realized and schizophrenia was a biological disease diagnosable by means of an objective test. Would a person suspected of having schizophrenia have the right to refuse to submit to such a test and thus be able to prevent being diagnosed as having schizophrenia?

* * *

One of the bitter ironies about current professional and popular attitudes concerning schizophrenia is that they rest on the unchallengeable assumption that, to cope effectively with the alleged disease, physicians must know its etiology. Unless the disease is contagious and thus presents a public health hazard, its cause is legally unimportant. In relation to schizophrenia, what is important is that both the law and psychiatry attribute homicide and suicide—and other socially disturbing behaviors—to "it." This is the motive and justification for the differences in the legal statuses of patients with schizophrenia and patients with epilepsy, multiple sclerosis, and Parkinsonism. (See also *Mental Illness*)

Science

Science is about truth and error.

Religion, politics, and psychiatry are about right and wrong, care and coercion.

* * *

In the nineteenth century, famous physicians did not look to Authority (Church/State) to validate their claims. They looked for it in their own minds and souls, in the opinion of their colleagues, and in the verdict of posterity. Their labors were not supported and were not corrupted by Authority, and the fruits of their labors often ran afoul of the untruths taught by Authority as truths. During the same period, famous psychiatrists looked to Authority (State/Law) to validate their claims. Their labors were supported and corrupted by Authority and the fruits of their labors formed an integral part of Authority's manufactory of official mendacity.

Today, most medical professionals look to Authority (State/Law) to validate their claims, are supported and corrupted by Authority, and their souls are no longer theirs. Cosseted by grants, titles, prizes, and access to Power, they are indifferent to the verdict of posterity (which they know or suspect will go against them).

Self

Self-centeredness and self-reliance, like fraternal twins, are closely related but are not identical.

Bringing up children, we must beware of pathologizing their self-centeredness, lest we inhibit their self-reliance.

Self-Control

Many people claim that they *cannot control themselves* and hence should not be held responsible for their (mis)behavior; for example, smokers, for their inability to control their craving for cigarettes; obese persons, for their inability to control their eating; promiscuous persons, for their inability to control their sexual urges; and so forth. Nevertheless, these persons expect to have the right to control others who *can control themselves*, by voting for politicians who deprive them of autonomy. (That there are no other kinds of politicians to vote for is another matter.)

Individuals who cannot control their cars are not accorded the privilege of working as driving instructors. Individuals who cannot control themselves should not be accorded the privilege of voting, much less being drug czars and presidents.

* * *

Many people fail in their elementary duty to control themselves, yet have the right to control others. *Mutatis mutandis*, many governments fail in their elementary duty to feed their own people, yet have the right to vote in the United Nations and thus influence the behavior of people on whose labor and largess they depend.

Governments that receive foreign aid ought not to be accorded the privilege of membership in the United Nations.

Self-Conversation

There are three ways in which we listen to a lecturer. 1) We listen closely and engage him in an ongoing inner dialogue, agree, or disagree with him. 2) We tune him out and engage in some private mental activity (daydream). 3) We become sleepy and perhaps doze off. I regard these options as evidence that we engage in ceaseless self-conversation.

* * *

People often value their belief in the "truth" of Judaism, Christianity, Marxism, or Mental Illness more highly than thinking clearly and fearlessly, that is, having a candid self-conversation.

Self-Esteem

Self-esteem is not something one can give another, like money. Much less is it something one can give oneself. Children have no reason to have self-esteem and *ought* to feel a lack of it.

Self-esteem rests on achievement and usefulness to others. Young children cannot do anything and have no reason to have self-esteem. As children mature, they may learn to do certain things better than their siblings, parents, teachers, or other adults. That will give them self-esteem.

Self-Improvement

The popularity of motivational speakers and other quacks peddling success and riches is interpreted as Americans' insatiable passion for self-improvement. Sadly, it is a symptom of just the opposite, of their insatiable lust for believing that there are easy answers to hard questions.

Sex

Love: The desire to merge lives.

Lust: The desire to merge bodies.

Two distinct elements that resist forming a stable compound, called "family"; once combined, prone to decombine in a process called "divorce."

* * *

Pornography is to sex as vulgarity is to language.

* * *

Sex therapist: Pimp and procurer with clinical credentials.

* * *

Infatuation: The name an observer gives to the condition of a man intensely attracted to a woman, or vice versa, when, according to the observer, the only thing the couple has in common is their sexual difference.

* * *

Marriage: 1. The desire to merge both bodies and lives—yielding, as a rule, the sacrifice of copulation for companionship or vice versa. 2. The state or condition of a community consisting of a husband, a wife, and two victims, making in all two. (*Pace* Ambrose Bierce.)

* * *

Masturbation: 1. Taking matters into one's own hands; formerly, medical authorities prohibited it, now they prescribe it. 2. The primary sexual activity of mankind: in the nineteenth century, a disease; in the twentieth, a cure.

* * *

One can teach a person to eat dietetically proper meals, but one cannot teach him to be a gourmet. Similarly, one can teach a person to perform sexually, but one cannot teach him to be erotic. Therein lies the absurdity of sex therapy.

* * *

There are two sexes. They could be called "complementary," but are called "opposites."

Sadly, this linguistic custom is more revealing of the true relations between the sexes than the entire lexicon of love.

* * *

One of the most powerful aphrodisiacs is the anticipation of erotic embrace with an absent beloved. It combines affection, lust, and novelty with the promise of fulfillment. The pleasurable exhilaration so generated is the very opposite of the dull and distasteful sensation of obligation engendered by the unremitting presence and availability of the partner, however beloved and sexually attractive.

* * *

Traditionally, men used power to gain sex, and women, sex to gain power. The new ethic of equality between men and women must come down to one of two things: either, as the romantics hope, that neither men nor women will use power to gain sex; or, as the realists expect, that both men and women will use power to gain sex, and sex to gain power.

* * *

Why is the sexual arousal and release of women more interesting—even for women—than the sexual arousal and release of men? Because the phenomenon is less obvious, leaving more to the imagination, which is the ultimate source of sexual excitement.

Secrecy of all kinds, epitomized by sexual secrecy, is a source of excitement demanding satisfaction.

* * *

Why do women fall in love? Because, explains Professor Gareth Leng of the University of Edinburgh, "a 'love potion' created in women's brains after the act of sex helps her to form a bond with her partner."[10]

Now we know why so many people are in love with themselves: Because they masturbate.

* * *

One cannot be an individual—a person separate from family and society—without having secrets.

Because secrets separate people, individualists treasure them and collectivists condemn them.

Keeping secrets separates people, sharing secrets unites them.

Confessing, gossiping, psychoanalysis, spying—each involves communicating secrets and thus establishing human relationships.

Traditionally, sex has been a private, secret activity. Therein lay part of its power for uniting individuals in a strong bond. As sexual activity becomes less secretive, we deprive it of some of its power to hold men and women together.

* * *

The pleasure of genital orgasm is the consequence of a well-articulated experience of controlled loss of control. This is why, in human societies, sex is both a brutalizing and a civilizing force.

* * *

Sexual desire may be a powerful impetus for bonding in animals but is a barrier to comfortable relations among human beings. (See also *Gender*)

Slavery

The essence of slavery is involuntary labor.

The essence of psychiatric slavery is involuntary treatment.

Cui bono? Who profits? Economically as well as existentially, the master, slaveholder: the involuntary labor of the slave benefited the plantation owner, the involuntary treatment of the mental patient benefits the psychiatrist.

Smoking

According to American and British physicians and governments, smoking is a disease. If so, it is a disease whose etiology, cigarettes, the state taxes and treats as an indispensable source of revenue. (The state does the same with the disease called "alcoholism," whose causative agent it taxes.)

* * *

The antismoking demagogues declare cigarettes to have no "valid uses." They deny that many people regard cigarettes as deodorants, perfumes, status symbols, tranquilizers, anti-obesity drugs, and the sources of existential comfort and physical pleasure.

Social Control

In the Christian world, people used to rely on religion and laws informed by religious myths as methods of social control. Now, they rely on psychiatry and laws informed by psychiatric myths.

In the Muslim world, people never exchanged social controls based on religion for social controls based on psychiatry.

Nowhere have people endeavored to fashion a society with social controls informed by the purely secular values of personal liberty and individual responsibility. In such a society, the law would not protect people from harming themselves, but would protect people from harm by others by not recognizing mental illness as an excuse.

Social Relations

The truth shall set us free, said Jesus. And lies unite us.

* * *

A person cannot make another happy, but he can make him unhappy. This is the main reason why there is more unhappiness than happiness in the world.

* * *

We appear unable or unwilling to accept the reality of human conflict. It is never simply man who offends against his fellow man: someone or something—the devil, mental illness, inequality, poverty—intervenes to obscure, excuse, and explain away man's terrifying inhumanity to man.

* * *

In science, it's dangerous to lie: if discovered, the liar is cast out of the group as a faker and fraud.

In religion, politics, and psychiatry, it's dangerous to tell the truth: if discovered, the truth-teller is cast out of the group as a heretic and a traitor.

* * *

The three monomanias of modern man: Monotheism, monogamy, and monomedicine.

* * *

Two wrongs don't make a right, but they make a good excuse.

* * *

When a person can no longer laugh at himself, it is time for others to laugh at him.

* * *

In Karl Marx and Sigmund Freud's vision, man is victim of oppression or repression. This vision supports the collectivist-totalitarian impulse to liberate man from the slavery of brutal capitalists and harsh superegos.

In Adam Smith and Ludwig von Mises's vision, man is a victor over instinct and impulse. This vision supports the individualist-libertarian dream of man controlling his own impulses and peacefully cooperating and coexisting with others.

* * *

Equality in human relations is like the ideal gas in physics. In real life, the most we can expect is mutually satisfying reciprocity. Ironically, this is hindered rather than hastened by striving for equality.

* * *

The natural state of mankind is poverty. Wealth is something we must create.

Similarly, the natural state of mankind is "mental illness": We begin life undisciplined, useless, and dependent, that is, "mentally ill." "Mental health"—as self-discipline, usefulness to others, and independence—is something we must create.

It is a mistake to think of poverty and mental illness as having "causes." It is an especially stupid mistake to think that mental illness causes poverty, or vice versa. Both are conditions that we must overcome, by personal effort.

* * *

No amount of religion and prayer can transform an undisciplined and uneducated peasant into an effective farmer producing a surplus of food.

Similarly, no amount of psychiatry and antipsychotic drugs can transform an undisciplined and uneducated youth into an effective person producing marketable goods or services.

* * *

Institutions such as chattel slavery and psychiatric slavery begin as solutions for social problems and become "problems" only much later.

Calling such arrangements "problems" implies that people are eager to eschew the benefits they derive from them, which is not true. Once it becomes true, the arrangement ceases to be an acceptable solution and is quickly abandoned.

This was the case, for example, with the practice of confining Japanese-Americans in so-called relocation camps, which stopped as soon as World War II ended. The fact that coercive psychiatric practices have become a chronic "social problem" suggests that it is not a problem that people are trying to solve.

* * *

All modern ideologies view certain classes of persons as *victims* of *oppression* and promise them *liberation*.

In communism, capitalists oppress workers; in feminism, men oppress women; in psychiatry/psychoanalysis, mental illness oppresses everyone.

What happens when the oppressed are liberated? Typically, the formerly oppressed claim non-responsibility for their inability to support themselves and demand that the state take care of them.

Workers expect the state to support them, by giving them jobs or welfare payments.

Women expect the state to pay for their abortions and care for their children.

Former mental patients expect the state to support them as mentally disabled and give them "services" that they control.

Socialism

Christianity without Jesus.

Speech

How does a psychiatrist or anyone else know that a person has delusions or hallucinates? He can know it only by hearing what the subject says. Absent speech by the subject, there can be no delusion or hallucination.

In short, delusions and hallucinations are speech acts. Hence, they ought to be protected by the First Amendment.

* * *

To a hearing person, a deaf-mute's hallucination, like his sign language, is a meaningless movement of his hands.

Standard of Care

In psychiatry, as in medicine, the profession determines what counts as the "standard of care" to which the psychiatrist must adhere in treating patients. "Where diagnostic and treatment procedures are appropriately documented in literature, a standard of medical care for a given disease entity or condition is applicable...the standards are rarely controversial..."[11]

If a psychiatrist deviates from "the applicable standard of care in his treatment of the patient," and the patient injures or kills himself or someone else, the psychiatrist will be found guilty of medical negligence.[12]

State

State monopoly of religion is the hallmark of the theological state.

State monopoly of medicine is the hallmark of the therapeutic state.

In theological and therapeutic states alike, the individual is deprived of autonomy, allegedly in his own best interest.

* * *

The welfare state seeks to relieve poverty and unemployment; its beneficiaries are not helped against their will; it is a constitutional state, regulated by the rule of law.

The therapeutic state seeks to remedy personal and social problems defined as diseases; its beneficiaries are often helped against their will; it is a totalitarian state, governed by the rule of therapeutic discretion.

* * *

It is an error to call the therapeutic state the "nanny state" or the "welfare state." Governesses control minors with the consent of their parents. Neither nannies nor social workers "treat" adults for nonexistent diseases against their will. Only psychiatrists have that power.

Statism

Conservatives use the state to prohibit people from doing what the conservatives deem is bad for them.

Liberals use the state to compel people to do what the liberals deem is good for them.

Psychiatrists use the state to do both: prohibit them from acting "psychotic" or killing themselves, by incarcerating them in insane asylums; and compel them to submit to treatment for the imaginary illnesses that allegedly cause these behaviors, by forcibly drugging them.

* * *

Statist policies lack the self-correcting mechanism of the market. That is why both command-economic and command-psychiatric forms of "assistance" are doomed to diminish the freedom and self-defined interests of their denominated beneficiaries.

Foreign aid and psychiatric funding alike augment the power and wealth of the bureaucrats who distribute and receive it, and exacerbate the miseries of the people they are supposed to benefit.

Sterilization, Mental

One of the meanings of the verb "to sterilize" is to deprive an animal or person of the power of reproduction (typically, by removal of the gonads or altering some part of the reproductive system).

- Pet owners often sterilize their cats or dogs. We call that "castration," "gelding," "neutering," or "spaying."
- Men sometimes choose to be sterilized by having their vas deferens ligated, and women by having their fallopian tubes tied. We call that "birth control" or "contraception."
- Certain dependents—retarded persons, mental patients, prisoners, political opponents deemed "degenerates"—are ordered to be sterilized by certain authorities, such as parents, physicians, legislators, judges. We call that "sterilization" or "forcible sterilization."

In each case, the aim of the sterilization is to improve the lives of those who authorize (and pay) for the procedure.

The hallucinations and delusions of schizophrenics resemble the pregnancy of retarded women unable to care for their infants. Engaging in sexual intercourse and becoming pregnant upsets the retarded woman's family and society, not the woman. "Hearing voices" upsets the schizophrenic patient's family and society, not the patient.

Formerly, retarded and mentally ill women were often sterilized without their consent or against their will. Today, psychotic patients are mentally sterilized without their consent or against their will: they are forcibly administered anti-schizophrenia drugs (or lobotomy or electric shock treatment) to eliminate or prevent hallucinations and delusions.

I interpret the fact that, when given an opportunity, most psychotic patients stop taking antipsychotic drugs as evidence that they are being mentally sterilized against their will and that their "treatment" benefits the patient's family, society, psychiatry, and the pharmaceutical industry, rather than the so-called patients themselves.

Stigma

In the Theological State, the worst stigma is being called a heretic.

In the Therapeutic State, the worst stigma is being called psychotic.

Suicide

Divorce from an unhappy marriage to life.

* * *

Breaking the habit of living.

* * *

Catholic dogma links suicide and murder, classifying both as grievous sins.

Psychiatric dogma also links suicide and murder, classifying both as serious sicknesses.

* * *

Threatening suicide: 1. A form of blackmail (intimidation by threatening auto-homicide instead of hetero-homicide). 2. A symptom of a severe mental illness, justifying coercive psychiatric intervention. 3. A weapon of the powerless against the powerful.

* * *

Dying voluntarily is a *choice* intrinsic to human existence. It is our ultimate, fatal freedom. However, that is not how the right-thinking person today sees voluntary death: he believes that no one in his right mind kills himself, that suicide is a mental health problem. Behind that belief lies a transparent evasion: relying on physicians to prevent suicide, prescribe suicide, and provide suicide—and thus avoid the subject of suicide. It is an evasion fatal to freedom.

* * *

We call the act of causing the death of a human being, by omission or commission, "homicide." Hence, suicide is a type of homicide.

Killing oneself differs radically from killing another person. The traditional, religion-inspired bracketing of self-murder with murder is, in our day, misleading.

To understand suicide, we must draw a clear distinction between it and murder: we ought to call killing oneself "autohomicide," and killing another person "heterohomicide."

* * *

Suicide: The sole escape from a life sentence. (Death by accident or illness is not willed and hence doesn't count.)

* * *

Suicide is to homicide as masturbation is to rape.

If we called killing oneself "auto-homicide," and killing others "hetero-homicide," we could better appreciate the distinction between these acts.

* * *

Suicide is to physician-assisted suicide as masturbation is to prostitute-assisted sex.

Suicide is to euthanasia without consent as masturbation is to rape.

Suicide is self-killing: regardless of what we call it, being killed by another person is not suicide.

* * *

Suicide is a fundamental human right. This does not mean that it is morally desirable. It means only that society does not have the moral right to interfere, by force, with a person's decision to commit this act.

* * *

Prohibiting what one cannot enforce degrades both authority and obedience, and undermines respect for both law and decency.

Prohibiting suicide is thus the ultimate folly, and the ultimate indecency.

* * *

He who does not accept and respect the choice to reject life does not truly accept and respect life itself.

* * *

Formerly, the person who killed himself was held responsible for his act and was punished for it. Now, his mental illness is held responsible for it and his psychiatrist is punished for having misdiagnosed and mistreated it.

* * *

Psychiatrists claim and many people apparently agree that suicide is a disease. However, suicide resembles a treatment more than a disease: it is the only effective remedy against what sometimes ails people, namely, the necessity to go on living.

* * *

As children grow up, they learn to what extent they are allowed and expected to take their lives into their own hands. The more they are allowed and expected to do so, the more likely they are to develop into autonomous, self-determining persons, who take not only their lives, but their deaths as well, into their own hands.

Persons who choose to be their own masters often also choose to be their own executioners.

* * *

The person who engages in behavior psychiatrists call a "suicidal gesture" or "suicidal threat" offends not because he wants to die, which is his inalienable right, but because he involves the public in what ought to be a private act. In short, his offense is that he is an exhibitionist.

Every man has an inalienable right to his penis, but no man has a right to exhibit it in public. Similarly, every man has an inalienable right to his intention to kill himself, but no man has the right to impose it on the public. The person who exhibits his intention to kill himself is indiscreet and indecorous, not insane.

* * *

In the ideology and jargon of psychiatry and law, a person labeled "severely mentally ill" is considered to be, *ipso facto*, "dangerous to himself and others."

This nonsensical phrase is used to justify involuntary psychiatric incarceration and "treatment" and is thus pivotal to the psychiatric enterprise.

Although it makes sense to say that a person is dangerous to others, it makes no sense to say that he is dangerous to himself (unless we assume, *a priori*, that he has two selves, one being dangerous to the other).

In fact, the person who wants to die differs from the person who wants to get rich only in his goal.

* * *

We call dying by disease "natural death," and dying by choice "suicide." Although in our political language we celebrate the value of autonomy, in our medical language we celebrate the value of heteronomy.

If we valued autonomy more, and dependence on medical authority less, we would call suicide "self-determined death."

* * *

The psychiatric prohibition of suicide—like the psychiatric prohibition of self-abuse (masturbation) and drug abuse (self-medication)—is emblematic of the culture's hostility to autonomy and of the psychiatrist's social function as agent of social control.

* * *

If a beloved and useful person kills himself, we dwell on the personal and economic loss his death causes.

If a despised and useless person kills himself, we deny the personal and economic gain that his death causes.

* * *

If Jones doesn't want to stay married, we don't consider it to be Smith's business to stop Jones from getting divorced.

If Jones doesn't want to go on living, why should it be Smith's business to keep him alive? What is there about being a psychiatrist that gives him the right, much less the duty, to prevent a person from killing himself?

Like being married, being alive is an opportunity, a challenge, a burden, in different proportions at different times.

Our customs, laws, and psychiatric practices with respect to suicide and suicide prevention reflect not our respect for life (as we like to pretend), but our fear of death and our passion to meddle in other people's lives.

* * *

During the past century, most people in developed countries concluded that when it comes to having children, less is more.

If we want to improve our lot on earth, we shall have to apply this principle to the length of our own life.

Having ten children is not necessarily better than having one or two. Why should living, say, ten more years at age seventy or eighty be better than living only five, two, one, or no more years?

We have learned that, to prosper as middle-aged persons, we must practice birth control when we are young.

We shall have to learn that, to prosper as old persons, we must practice death control while we can.

* * *

By definition, suicide is a type of homicide—the killing of a human being. We recognize that killing another person is a morally, psychologically, and socially complex phenomenon: the law distinguishes first-degree murder, second-degree murder, voluntary manslaughter, involuntary manslaughter, homicide in self-defense, and so forth.

We refuse to recognize that killing oneself is an equally complex phenomenon: the law recognizes only two kinds of self-killings, suicide committed while sane and suicide committed while insane.

* * *

To be accountable or responsible for preventing his patient's suicide, the psychiatrist would have to wield far-reaching powers over the patient's capacity to act.

In practice, it is virtually impossible to prevent the suicide of a person determined on killing himself.

Coercive psychiatric interventions to prevent suicide deprive the patient of liberty and dignity. Their use is both impractical and immoral.

* * *

Some people believe that a person should have a right to kill himself: that criminal and mental health laws regarding the intention, alleged intention, or attempt to kill oneself ought to be abolished.

Others believe that a person should have a right to physician-assisted suicide and euthanasia: that laws prohibiting the physician from deliberately killing a patient ought, sometimes, to be suspended.

I support the right to suicide but not the right to physician-assisted suicide. Physician-assisted suicide gives a right to physicians that belongs to patients; it fosters medical-statist tutelage, not self-determination and self-responsibility.

* * *

Films, television programs, and the print media inundate Americans with messages that, in effect, show them how to kill others. Yet, Americans are rarely shown how to kill themselves.

Clearly, we are attracted to murder and love to hear and see how it's done, but are afraid of, or repelled by, suicide and don't want to hear or see how to it's done.

What this tells us about ourselves I leave to the reader to decide.

* * *

So massive and mindless is the fear of suicide, especially among physicians, that many endorse euthanasia, justifying killing their "hopelessly ill" patients with the rationalization that "if we don't help them to die, they will kill themselves."

* * *

In September 1987, the delegates of the California Bar Association "approved legislation that would allow physicians to give terminally ill patients a prescription for a legal dose of drugs.... A psychiatrist would have to certify that the patient was rational."[13]

In the theological state, clerics held the keys to the Kingdom of Heaven.

In the therapeutic state, clinicians hold the keys to the Kingdom of Death.

The elemental human cry seems to be: "Give me parents, give me priests, give me doctors, give me any authority to control me, but don't give me autonomy—don't leave me alone!"

* * *

In language and logic we are the prisoners of our premises, just as in politics and law we are the prisoners of our rulers. Hence, we had better pick them well. For if suicide is an illness because it terminates in death and if the prevention of death by any means necessary is the physician's therapeutic mandate, then the proper remedy for suicide is liberticide.

* * *

We are born involuntarily, to please (or displease) others. That is what makes dying voluntarily the ultimate freedom; why religion and psychiatry insist that we ought to die involuntarily; and why dying voluntarily is the ultimate heresy and madness—lèse majesté against religion and medicine, church and state.

* * *

Americans differ about whether practicing contraception is right or wrong. Still, most Americans agree that the decision to practice birth control or abstain from the practice is a choice that American men and women ought to be able to make without help or hindrance by physicians and without interference by the state.

Our attitude toward practicing death control ought to be the same. Not until we are free to make decisions about death control without help or hindrance by the state will we be in formal possession of our most basic freedom—the freedom to decide when and how we die.

* * *

We collectively approve of birth control; hence, we do not automatically impugn a person's competence to practice contraception and do not try to interfere with his behavior on the ground that he is not competent to decide about so vital a matter.

We collectively disapprove of death control (suicide); hence, we automatically impugn a person's competence to practice death control and interfere coercively with his behavior on precisely that ground.

* * *

Vases made of glass are more fragile than vases made of steel. The lives of lonely and depressed persons are more fragile than the lives of persons engaged in life and who are not depressed. The "condition" psychiatrists call "being suicidal" is and ought to be regarded as a disposition: some people are more likely to kill themselves than others, just as some vases are more likely to break than others.

From a relatively early age, every person can imagine killing himself and is, in a manner of speaking, "suicidal." A person disposed to kill himself knows that he is so disposed. If he wants to protect himself from his inclination, he can do so by avoiding objects or situations that would facilitate his self-destruction or by asking others to protect him.

The person who undertakes the complex task of killing himself is responsible for his premeditated act, just as the person who undertakes to carry out any other complex task is responsible for executing it.

One of psychiatry's most fundamental mandates and most far-reaching confusions stems from the belief that it is the psychiatrist's job to prevent "suicidal" persons from killing themselves.

* * *

When a person under psychiatric care kills himself, he is invariably referred to as a "suicidal patient" whose death ought to have been prevented. This is confusing hindsight with foresight. Being suicidal is a disposition. Committing suicide is an action. Since the act can be performed only once, we cannot know whether it is the result of a disposition or the result of a unique decision.

We do not call a respected rabbi or judge or physician (with no criminal record) who suddenly kills his wife "homicidal." On the contrary, we express astonishment that he has engaged in such behavior. Committing murder is a discrete action; it may or may not be the manifestation of a disposition.

Unless a person tells his psychiatrist that he plans to kill himself and the psychiatrist records that information, there is no way of ascertaining whether a person who has killed himself was or was not "suicidal." All that we know about such an individual is that he has killed himself. Calling all such persons "suicidal" after the fact, and every person who kills another "homicidal" after the fact, are tautologies masquerading as explanations.

* * *

If you cut off your penis, psychiatrists say you have a mental illness and lock you up in a mental hospital. But if psychiatrists say you have transsexualism and you give consent to a surgeon to cut off your penis, then you are receiving treatment for an illness.

If you cut off your life, psychiatrists say you did it because you were mentally ill. If you try to cut off your life and fail, psychiatrists say you are mentally ill and dangerous to yourself and lock you up in a mental hospital. If the state cuts off your life, you are receiving capital punishment.

If you request a physician to cut off your life, and if psychiatrists approve your request, then you are receiving "physician-assisted suicide" (PAS), a form of killing that the advocates of PAS want to add to the repertoire of medical treatments.

* * *

If a prisoner condemned to death kills himself, we recognize his act as deliberate and rational and say: "He has cheated the hangman."

If a man condemned to debility, disease, helplessness, hopelessness, old age, and other miseries kills himself, we don't recognize his act as deliberate and rational, and say: "His depression was undiagnosed and he died needlessly; his untreated depression killed him."

Paying homage to this false explanation as scientific truth is the fee a person must pay to gain entry into the official discourse of psychiatry and mental health policy.

* * *

I wish neither to praise and recommend, nor condemn and discourage suicide. I am simply saying that:

- We have a choice, and hence a responsibility, between staying the course, living until death claims us, or quitting before it does, by killing ourselves.

- This choice-and-responsibility is, in principle, similar to the choice-and-responsibility for staying single and getting married, staying childless and having children, and so forth.

- *We ought to debate and resolve the problem of physician-prevented suicide before we engage in debating or legislating about physician-provided suicide.*

Suicide is goal-directed behavior for which the actor has reasons and for which he, and he alone, is responsible. Medical considerations are as irrelevant to killing oneself as they are to killing others.

Suicide Prevention

The priest is prevented by his oath of secrecy from denouncing the suicidal penitent to the health authorities.

The lawyer is prevented by his code of professional conduct from denouncing the suicidal client to the health authorities: "Suicide is not a crime in New York and under its applicable ethical rules, a lawyer may not disclose apparent or inferred 'intentions' to commit suicide."[14]

The psychiatrist is mandated—by the ethical code of his profession, the "standard of psychiatric care," and the law—to denounce the suicidal patient to the health authorities and imprison ("hospitalize") him.

* * *

Preventing people from killing themselves is a basic medical and moral mandate of the psychiatrist.

Killing oneself is a choice and hence an expression of one's personal freedom. Forcibly interfering with that freedom is, *by definition*, a deprivation of liberty.

* * *

There is no evidence that hospitalizing a person against his will to prevent him from killing himself is an effective method for preventing his suicide.

Who, then, benefits from this practice? The persons who initiate the action, typically, the patient's relatives.

* * *

We have rid ourselves of the false beliefs that individuals who practice contraception, masturbation, or homosexuality are depraved or diseased and have effectively barred the state and its psychiatric agents from interfering with persons who engage in such behaviors.

I feel confident that the time will come when people will look back at our present prohibitory policies toward suicide with the same amazed disapproval with which we look back at our past prohibitory policies toward contraception, masturbation, and homosexuality.

T

Theory

Scientists use the term "theory" to *explain natural phenomena*, for example, the transmission of heat and light from the sun to the earth.

Lawyers use it to *justify social policies*, for example, chattel slavery, university admission quotas, or, as the following example illustrates, animal rights: "Harvard Law School professor [Steven M.] Wise...[is] trying to develop legal theories to advance his cause...breaching the legal wall that separates humans from nonhumans."[1]

Therapeutic State

"Although we may not know it, we have, in our day, witnessed the birth of the Therapeutic State. This is perhaps the major implication of psychiatry as an institution of social control."[2]

* * *

Prior to World War II, the American system of social controls rested on Christian moral values and was enforced by a judicial apparatus based on English common law, the Constitution, and the rule of law. Since then, our system of social controls has become increasingly dependent on the principles of a politicized medicine, and has been legitimized and enforced by a complex state apparatus that commingles the principles and practices of paternalistic "therapy," punitive psychiatry, collectivistic public health, and the criminal justice system. To articulate this insight, I proposed three new terms.

In 1960 I coined the phrase "myth of mental illness," to dramatize that neither diagnoses nor behaviors are diseases.[3]

In 1963, I proposed the term "therapeutic state" to identify the transformation of our dominant political ideology from a democratic welfare state legitimized by the rule of law into an autocratic therapeutic state legitimized by psychiatry as a branch of medicine.[4]

In 1974 I coined the term "pharmacracy," to identify the use of medical methods in the service of political rule and social control, not medical healing.[5]

* * *

The theological state was characterized by monoconfessional religious regulations.

The therapeutic state is characterized by monomedical pharmacratic regulations.[6]

* * *

In the theological state, people are obsessed with religion, salvation, and heresy.

In the therapeutic state, people are obsessed with health, treatment, and quackery.

When religion and the state are separated, heresy loses its political-legal significance: it becomes a parochial issue for a particular sect, its officials and members.

Were medicine and the state separated, quackery would lose its political-legal significance: it would become a parochial issue for a particular system of healing, its practitioners and followers.

The unlikeliness of the latter prospect is a manifestation of the intensity of our reliance on the state for the protection of our bodies, a dependence analogous to our ancestors' dependence on the church for the protection of their souls.

* * *

Missionary clerics define natives as "heathens" and feel it is their duty to "save" them.

Missionary clinicians define people as "patients" and feel it is their duty to cure them.

* * *

We have exchanged theobabble for psychobabble and call it "progress," "science," and "therapy."

* * *

For the Hasid, the pious Jew, God's rules permeate all of life, leaving no behavior exempt from religious scrutiny and the proper observance of religious duties.

We have become medical Hasidim: medical rules permeate all of life, leaving no behavior exempt from medical scrutiny and the proper observance of medical duties.

* * *

The term "treatment" is the grand legitimizer of our age. Call your effort or intention "treatment," and presto—you are a great humanitarian and scientist.

Sigmund Freud called listening and talking to his voluntary patients "treatment"—and psychoanalysis is now recognized as a form of medical treatment.

Ugo Cerletti gave his involuntary patients electrically induced convulsions and called the torture "treatment"—and electroshock is now recognized as a form of medical treatment.

William Masters hired women to copulate with men and called it "sex therapy"—and sex therapy is now recognized as a form of medical treatment.

* * *

In 1966, an international team of public health physicians declared that the task of the medical profession "is to bring about a change in day-to-day behavior, to create a new style of life...*a new morality.* The aims of such an education would include sound child-rearing practices, a balanced life style, rational dietary habits, the elimination or reduction of the consumption of certain modern toxic substances such as tobacco or alcohol."[7]

Virtually everything the Founding Fathers sought to achieve by separating church and state has been undone by the apostles of modern medicine, whose zeal for creating a therapeutic state has remained unopposed by politicians, priests, professionals, journalists, civil libertarians, and the public.

* * *

In a capitalist state, a person ought to be able to obtain narcotics in exchange for money. In a therapeutic state, he can obtain narcotics only in exchange for pain, and often not even then.

* * *

Capitalism generates the production of goods and services; therapeutism, the production of diseases and treatments.

* * *

In a therapeutic society, medical services are free, but people are not; in an open society, people are free, but nothing else is.

* * *

Conservatives want to make people virtuous; liberals want to make them healthy. Both believe that using the state to accomplish their aim is legitimate. That is why both conservatives and liberals favor anti-drug laws, psychiatric coercions, and other assaults against individual freedom and responsibility couched in therapeutic terms.

* * *

Two hundred years ago, the government of the United States was established on the principle that there are certain things it *must not do* to the people. These injunctions are properly called the Bill of Rights.

Today, the government of the United States is founded on the principle that there are certain things it *must do for or to* the people. These prescriptions ought properly to be called the Bill of Wrongs.

* * *

What the Sharia is to the Islamic State, the Diagnostic and Statistical Manual of the American Psychiatric Association is to the therapeutic state.

* * *

In a theocratic state, the government does not teach people religion; it forces them to believe the official theological falsehoods and silences the skeptics.

In a therapeutic state, the government does not teach people health; it forces them to believe the official therapeutic falsehoods and silences the skeptics.

* * *

Americans now expect physicians and other medical personnel to bring them into the world; teach them how to live; cure them when they fall ill; prevent them from harming themselves or others; and kill them when they are old.

The more physicians fulfill these expectations, the unhappier people, as patients, become with the medical profession.

Why? Because the patient's expectations are fulfilled on terms set by physicians and the state, not on terms set by the patient.

* * *

When a child in a family of Christian Scientists dies without medical attendance, say of diabetes, his parents are prosecuted for child-neglect or manslaughter.

At the same time, the Federal Government recognizes Christian Science as a legitimate method of healing. The 1989 edition of *The Medicare Handbook* states: "Medical hospital insurance can help pay for inpatient hospital and skilled nursing facility services you receive in a participating Christian Science sanatorium if it is operated or listed and certified by the First Church of Christ, Scientist, in Boston."[8]

Revealingly, this passage, headed "Care in a Christian Science Sanatorium," appears on the same page as the passage headed "Care in a Psychiatric Hospital."

Having assumed the role of determining what is, and what is not, legitimate medical treatment, the American government has decreed that faith healing is on a par with scientific-medical treatment, abolishing the fundamental distinction between ceremonial and technical healing.

* * *

Literary anticipations of the therapeutic state and its pharmacratic system of social controls:

Lord Byron

> This is the patent-age of new inventions / For killing bodies, and for saving souls, / All propagated with the best intentions.[9]

Samuel Butler

> As I have already said, these [persons we regard as criminals], though not judicially punishable, are recognized as requiring correction. Accordingly, there exists a class of men trained in soul-craft, whom they call straighteners, as nearly as I can translate a word which literally means "one who bends back the crooked."... Indeed, the straighteners have gone so far as to give names from the hypothetical language (as taught at the College of Unreason) to all known forms of mental indisposition, and to classify them according to a system of their own, which, though I could not understand it, seemed to work well in practice; for they are always able to tell a man what is the matter with him as soon as they have heard his story, and their familiarity with the long names assures him that they thoroughly understand his case.... I have never heard of a reasonable Erewhonian refusing to do what his straightener told him, any more than of a reasonable Englishman refusing to undergo even the most frightful operation if his doctors told him it was necessary."[10]

> No more swearing. No more bad language of any kind. A lamb-like temper ensured in about twenty minutes, by a single dose of one of our spiritual indigestion tabloids. In cases of all the more ordinary moral ailments, from simple lying to homicidal mania, in cases again of tendency to hatred, malice, and uncharitableness; or atrophy of the sympathetic instincts, etc., our spiritual indigestion tabloids will afford unfailing and immediate relief.[11]

Butler wrote this more than 150 years before Welsh psychiatrist David Healy, author of *The Creation of Psychopharmacology*, hailed the "discovery of Thorazine [as] significant in the history of medicine as the discovery of penicillin," and stated that "in their short lifespan they [antipsychotic drugs] have revolutionized psychiatry."[12]

H. G. Wells

> "[T]here was no such concentration of authority in their world [explains Urthred, a member of the new society]. In the past there had been, but it had long since diffused back into the general body of the community. *Decisions in regard to any particular matter were made by people who knew most about that matter.*"
>
> "But suppose [asks Mr. Cecil Burleigh, the visiting 'earthling'] it is a decision that has to be generally observed? A rule affecting the public health? Who would enforce it?"
>
> "It would not need to be enforced. Why should it?"
>
> "But suppose someone refused to obey your regulation?"
>
> "We should inquire why he or she did not conform. There might be some exceptional reason."
>
> "But failing that?"
>
> "We should make an inquiry into his mental and moral health."
>
> *"The mind doctor takes the place of the policeman," said Mr. Burleigh....*
>
> *"The activities of our world," said Urthred, "are all coordinated to se-*

cure the general freedom."[13]

The essence of pharmacracy lies precisely in such equating of freedom with medical-psychiatric control.

C. S. Lewis

[I]t is the function of the Conditioners to control.... They know how to *produce* conscience and decide what kind of conscience they will produce. They themselves are outside, above.… I am not supposing them to be bad men. They are, rather, not men (in the old sense) at all. They are, if you like, men who have sacrificed their own share in traditional humanity in order to devote themselves to the task of deciding what "Humanity" shall henceforth mean. "Good" and "bad" applied to them are words without content: for it is from them that the content of these words is henceforth to be derived.... [T]heir subjects [are not] necessarily unhappy men. They are not men at all: they are artifacts. Man's final conquest has proved to be the abolition of Man….[14]

Of all the tyrannies a tyranny sincerely exercised for the good of the victims may be the most oppressive…. To be "cured" against one's will and cured of states which we may not even regard as disease is to be put on a level with those who have not yet reached the age of reason or those who never will; to be classed with infants, imbeciles, and domestic animals.[15]

Aldous Huxley

In the Brave New World of my fable there was no whisky, no tobacco, no illicit heroin, no bootlegged cocaine. People neither smoked, nor drank, nor sniffed, nor gave themselves injections. Whenever anyone felt depressed or below par, he would swallow a tablet or two of a chemical compound called soma.... [T]he soma habit was not a private vice; it was a political institution, it was the very essence of Life, Liberty, and the Pursuit of Happiness guaranteed by the Bill of Rights. But this most precious of the subject's inalienable privileges was at the same time one of the most powerful instruments of rule in the dictator's armory. The systematic drugging of individuals for the benefit of the State.[16]

Adolfo Bioy Casares

Epitaph for the therapeutic state:

Well then, maybe it would be worth mentioning the three periods of history. When man believed that happiness was dependent upon God, he killed for

> religious reasons. When he believed that happiness was dependent upon the form of government, he killed for political reasons.... After dreams that were too long, true nightmares...we arrived at the present period of history. Man woke up, discovered that which he always knew, that happiness is dependent upon health, and began to kill for therapeutic reasons.... When no one believed any longer in the politicians, it was medicine, with its amazing discoveries, that captured the imagination of the human race. It is medicine that has come to replace both religion and politics in our time.[17]

Time

Time is not something we *have*, like money, and can exchange for something else we *want.* Time is a kind of "space" in which we *live*.

The adage, "If you want something done, ask a busy man to do it," expresses that wisdom.

* * *

We say we *have* time, *spend* time, *serve* time, *waste* time; that time *passes* quickly or slowly, *hangs* heavily, *disappears*, and so forth.

But time is not like money, of which we have much or little, of which some have more than others.

Time, like death, is the great equalizer. We all have the same amount of time: one lifetime, per person. The question is not how to spend time, but how to live life.

* * *

Time is an existential commodity of which there is always either a glut or a scarcity. The young and the old have too much time on their hands.

The young waste time, deluding themselves that its passage alone will turn them into adults.

The middle-aged have too little time, feeling perpetually harassed, trying to keep up in the proverbial rat race.

The old wait out time, deluding themselves that not dying is living.

Timidity

The most powerful friend of religion; the most powerful foe of individual liberty and personal responsibility; the reason why most people never grow up.

Transsexualism

Transsexualism as disease was invented in 1953 by Harry Benjamin, M.D., a German-born endocrinologist practicing in New York.

Considered the "father of transsexualism," Benjamin maintained that transsexualism is a bona fide disease because: "What both treatments [insulin for diabetes, sex-reassignment surgery for transsexualism] accomplish is the preservation of the life of the patient. Otherwise, many of these people would commit suicide."[18]

The insulin-deprived diabetic dies of diabetes.

The surgery-deprived transsexual does not—indeed *cannot*—die of transsexualism.

* * *

If we accept Benjamin's logic for classifying transsexualism as a disease, we would have to classify many displeasurable situations as diseases if the affected persons threaten to kill themselves unless their "medical" demands are met.

An old person threatens to kill himself unless a plastic surgeon makes him look younger: Would that make his displeasurable condition a disease called "transchronologicalism"?

A "psychotic" person threatens to kill himself unless an ophthalmologist removes his eyes: Would that make his displeasurable condition a disease called "transvisualism"?

Treat, Treatment

The verb "treat" can be used in the sense of "consider as" or "deal with," or in the sense of "intervene to remedy a disease."

Treat a solid as a liquid, but it will not behave as a liquid.

Treat a healthy person as a tuberculosis patient, but he will not have tuberculosis.

Treat a healthy person as a neurological patient, but he will not have a neurological disease.

Treat a healthy person as a mental patient, and he will have a mental disease.

* * *

Whether X has a bodily illness (tuberculosis) does not depend on whether we believe that he has such an illness. But whether X has a mental illness (schizophrenia) does depend on whether we believe that he has such a disease.

* * *

Treatment: 1. Intervention sought by a patient from a physician for the amelioration or cure of disease. 2. Punishment, as in "Let's give him the treatment..."; especially popular in psychiatric institutions and totalitarian countries.

* * *

Free trade in drugs—such as barbiturates, chloral hydrate, and opiates—is prohibited, depriving people of the pharmacological tools necessary for committing suicide effectively and painlessly.

Instead of seeking repeal of drug prohibition, many people advocate "physician-assisted" suicide, that is, physicians writing prescriptions for lethal drugs. Timothy E. Quill and his collaborators call this medical bootlegging of barbiturates "an extraordinary and irreversible *treatment.*"[19]

Truth

Jesus said: "The truth shall set you free." He did not say: "The truth shall make you happy."

* * *

The truth shall set you free. The lie shall make you feel secure.

* * *

The truth may be painful, the lie, comforting; that doesn't make truth-telling bad and lying good.

* * *

To truth belongs knowledge, to error, belief.

V

Value

If you don't value your family, you will not have a family that values you.

If you don't value money or health or liberty, you will have no money or health or liberty.

If you don't value knowledge and competence and self-reliance, no one, including yourself, will value you—and no amount of psychiatric treatment will remedy your failure to value what is worthy.

Violence

Classifying both murder and suicide as violence, and treating both as problems in public health and psychiatry, is one of the doctrinal foundations of the therapeutic state.

According to a 2002 report by the World Health Organization, "Violence kills more than 1.6 million people each year, and suicide claims almost as many lives as war and homicide combined."[1]

Classifying murder and suicide as members of the same class of behaviors, called "violence," is like classifying taxation and philanthropy, stealing and gifting as members of the same class of behaviors, called "wealth transfer."

W

War

Formerly, we fought wars against nations and the aim was to win.

Today, we fight wars against terrorism and the aim is to "degrade" the adversary's ability to aid "terrorists."

Y

Youth

The principal tasks of youth: developing self-discipline and acquiring marketable skills.

Z

Zombification

The result of successful somatic treatment of mental illness.

Zoophobia Psychiatrica

The mental patient's (realistic) fear of the "wild-beast" psychiatrist, bent on "treating" him against his will.

Notes

A

1. Robin Norwood, quoted in "Getting beyond Mr. Wrong," *San Francisco Chronicle*, February 26, 1988, p. E14.
2. Ronald D. Laing, *The Politics of Experience and the Bird of Paradise* (Harmondsworth: Penguin, 1967), pp. 118-119.
3. Ronald D. Laing, *The Divided Self: An Existential Study in Sanity and Madness* (London: Tavistock Publications, 1960), p. 27, emphasis added.
4. John Clay, *R. D. Laing: A Divided Self* (London: Hodder & Stoughton, 1996), p. 181. See also Clancy Sigal, *Zone of the Interior* (New York: Popular Library, 1978).
5. David Cooper, *The Dialectics of Liberation* (Harmondsworth: Penguin, 1968), p. 7.
6. Michel Foucault, *Mental Illness and Psychology* [1954], translated by Alan Sheridan (New York: Harper Colophon, 1976), pp. 26, 28.
7. Quoted in Roger Kimball, "The perversions of Michel Foucault," *The New Criterion*, Vol. 11, No. 7, March 1993. http://www.newcriterion.com/archive/11/mar93/foucault.htm
8. Roger Kimball, "The perversions of Michel Foucault," *The New Criterion*, ibid.
9. Ronald D. Laing, *The Politics of Experience and the Bird of Paradise* (Harmondsworth: Penguin, 1967); David Cooper, *The Death of the Family* (New York: Pantheon, 1970).
10. Peter R. Breggin, "Empathic self-transformation and love in individual and family therapy," *The Humanistic Psychologist*, 27: 267-282 (Autumn), 1999.
11. Thomas Szasz, "Some observations on the use of tranquilizing agents," *A.M.A. Archives of Neurology and Psychiatry*, 77: 86-92 (January), 1957; p. 91.
12. John Carey, "A missionary zeal," *The Sunday Times Books* (London), February 23, 2003, pp. 35-36.
13. Quoted in, "A President for All Americans?" *Austin American-Statesman*, May 19, 1990, p. A21.
14. Paul Kurtz, "The growth of antiscience," *Skeptical Inquirer,* 18: 255-267, (Spring), 1994.
15. Anthony de Jasay, *Against Politics: On Government, Anarchy, and Order* (London: Routledge, 1997), p. 219.

B

1. Daniel R. Weinberger, "A brain too young for good judgment" (Op-Ed), *New York Times*, March 10, 2001.
2. Thomas Szasz, "Anatomy of a teenage shooting" (Letter), *New York Times*, March 13, 2001, Internet edition.
3. *Griswold v. Connecticut*, 381 U.S. 479, 1965.

4. The Swartz Foundation, "More about the mind/brain lecture series," emphasis added; http://www.stonybrook.edu/sb/mind/lectureseries.shtml; http://www.swartzneuro.org/index2.cfm
5. Michael Polanyi, "Life's Irreducible Structures" [1968], in Michael Polanyi, *Knowing and Being*, edited by Marjorie Grene (Chicago: University of Chicago Press, 1968), p. 238.
6. Werner Heisenberg, *Physics and Philosophy: The Revolution in Modern Science* (New York: Harper & Row, 1958), pp. 106, 199.
7. Hippocrates, "On the Sacred Disease (Epilepsy)," from *The Genuine Works of Hippocrates,* translated from the Greek by Francis Adams (Robert E. Krueger Publishing Co., Huntington, N.Y. 1972). http://www.humanistictexts.org/hippocrates.htm

C

1. *NAMI E-News,* March 13, 2001, Vol. 01-83, emphasis added.
2. John S. Werry, "Child psychiatric disorders: Are they classifiable?" *British Journal of Psychiatry*, 161: 472-480, 1992; p. 478, emphasis added.
3. American Psychiatric Association, *Diagnostic and Statistical Manual of Mental Disorders, DSM-III* (Washington, D.C.: American Psychiatric Association, 1980), pp. 63-64.
4. David Fassler, "Treatment for children" (Letters), *New York Times*, January 21, 2003. http://www.nytimes.com/2003/01/21/opinion/L21DRUG.html

D

1. Jim Bolton, "How can we reduce the stigma of mental illness?" *British Medical Journal*, 326: 357 (February 22), 2003. http://bmj.com/cgi/content/full/326/7386/S57a?eaf
2. Jerry Seper, "U.S. rearrest rate leapt to 67 percent in 1994," *Washington Times*, June 3, 2002; "Recidivism of Prisoners Released in 1994," June 2, 2002, Bureau of Justice Statistics, U.S. Department of Justice. http://www.washingtontimes.com/national/20020603-23068876.htm
3. See Shankar Vedantam, "Against depression, a sugar pill is hard to beat: Placebos improve mood, change brain chemistry in majority of trials of antidepressants," *Washington Post*, May 7, 2002; Page A01. http://www.washingtonpost.com/wp-dyn/articles/A42930-2002May6.html
4. David Levering Lewis, "An American pastime," *New York Review of Books*, November 21, 2002, pp. 27-30; p. 27.
5. Zannah Lewis, "Prozac has cats feline better," Birmingham Post (UK), April 4, 2003. http://icbirmingham.icnetwork.co.uk/0100news/0100localnews/page.cfm?objectid=12808314&method=full
6. Harry Anderson et al., "The global poison trade," *Newsweek*, November 7, 1988, pp. 66-68; p. 68.
7. Partnership for a Drug-Free America, "Sometimes..." (Advertisement), *Newsweek*, April 11, 1988.
8. Sally Satel, "For addicts, force is the best medicine," *Wall Street Journal*, January 7, 1998, p. 6.
9. Revelations, 13:10. *The Holy Bible*, Revised Standard Version (New York: Meridian, 1964), p. 235.
10. This attribution is apocryphal. See Tom Burnam, *The Dictionary of Misinformation* (New York: Ballantine Books, 1975), pp. 129-130.

11. Samuel Butler, *Erewhon* [1872] (Harmondsworth: Penguin, 1954), p. 193.

E

1. Quoted in Alan Ebenstein, *Friedrich Hayek: A Biography* (New York: Palgrave, 2001), p. 261.
2. Thomas Jefferson, *Notes on the State of Virginia* [1781], in Adrienne Koch and William Peden, editors, *The Life and Selected Writings of Thomas Jefferson* (New York: Modem Library, 1944), p. 276.
3. Immanuel Kant, quoted in Isaiah Berlin, *Four Essays on Liberty* (London: Oxford University Press 1969), p. 137.
4. Barbara W. Tuchman, "A nation in decline?" *New York Times Magazine*, September 20, 1987, pp. 52-56, 142-145; p. 142.
5. Thomas Szasz, *Law, Liberty, and Psychiatry: An Inquiry Into the Social Uses of Mental Health Practices* (New York: Macmillan, 1963), pp. 3-4.
6. G. Brock Chisholm, "The psychiatry of enduring peace and social progress," *Psychiatry*, 9: 3-11 (January), 1946; p. 9.

G

1. Daniel Goleman, "Biology of brain may hold key for gamblers: When the casino becomes an addiction, the condition may be chemical," *New York Times*, October 3, 1989, p. C1.
2. Quoted in Bill Stokes, "Gambling is being treated as a disease," *Buffalo News*, March 29, 1988, p. C7.
3. J. H. Tanne, "Paradise now: Picturing the genetic revolution," *British Medical Journal*, 321: 903 (October 7), 2000.

H

1. Quoted in Sidney and Beatrice Webb, *Soviet Communism: A New Civilisation* (2 vols.; New York: Charles Scribner's, 1938), vol. 2, p. 836.

I

1. William James, *The Principles of Psychology* [1890] (New York: Dover, 1950), vol. 1, p. 293.
2. Linda Villarosa, "Race: Scientists say it doesn't exist, so why don't we get over it?" (New York Times News Service), *The Post-Standard* (Syracuse), January 14, 2002, p. A-8.
3. Marcus Aurelius, "Brainy Quotes," http://webpdp.gator.com/v3/webpdp_v3_plugin.php?yic=HIC_L90DT
4. Sir Hartley Shawcross, *Trial of the Major War Criminals Before the International Military Tribunal*, Nuremberg, Germany. Proceedings, 19 July-29 July 1946, Vol. XIX, July 26, 1946, p. 467.
5. "North's motivation irrelevant, prosecutors say," *Syracuse Herald Journal*, March 8, 1989, p. A4.
6. Arnold W. Green, "The reified villain," *Social Research*, 35: 686-664 (Winter), 1963; p. 664.
7. See Karl Menninger, *The Crime of Punishment* (New York: Viking, 1968); Thomas Szasz, *Insanity: The Idea and Its Consequences* [1987] (Syracuse: Syracuse University Press, 1997).

J

1. Quoted in E. S. Turner, "The accoucheur's son," *Times Literary Supplement*, March 23, 2001, p. 36.

K

1. Norbert Wiener, *Ex-Prodigy: My Childhood and Youth* (New York: Simon and Schuster, 1953), p.144.

L

1. Aristotle, *De Poetica* (Poetics), translated by Ingram Bywater, in Richard McKean, editor, *The Basic Works of Aristotle* (New York: Random House, 1941), p. 1479.
2. Henry John Temple Palmerston (1784-1865), British foreign secretary, home secretary, and prime minister; quoted in Roland N. Stromberg, *Arnold J. Toynbee: History for an* Age *in Crisis* (Carbondale, Illinois Southern Illinois University Press, 1972), p. 102.
3. C. S. Lewis, *The Abolition of Man* [1947] (New York: Macmillan, 1967), p. 85, emphasis in the original.
4. William F. Buckley, Jr., "'To be a pilgrim': A visit to Lourdes," *National Review*, August 9, 1993, pp. 33-40; p. 40.
5. Ronald D. Laing, quoted in http://www.zatang.com/categories/literature/\bookreview/ajai/bookreview.htm
6. George Steiner, *Language and Silence: Essays on Language, Literature and the Inhuman* (New York: Athenaeum, 1967), p. 123.
7. Winfred Overholser, "Statement," in *Constitutional Rights of the Mentally Ill*. Hearings before the Subcommittee on Constitutional Rights of the Committee of the Judiciary, United States Senate, Eight-seventh Congress, First Session. Part I - Civil Aspects. March 28, 29 and 30, 1961 (Washington, D.C.: U.S. Government Printing Office, 1961), p. 38, emphasis added.
8. Quoted in Jean Orieux, *Voltaire,* translated by Barbara Bray and Helen R. Lane (Garden City, NY: Doubleday, 1979), p. 284.
9. Milton Friedman, *Capitalism and Freedom* (Chicago: University of Chicago Press, 1962), p. 15.
10. Plato, *Apology*, 38a.
11. C. S. Lewis, *The Abolition of Man* [1947] (New York: Macmillan, 1967).
12. Editorial, "The advertising of cigarettes," *JAMA*, 138: 652 (October 30), 1948.
13. Gabriel Josipovici, *The Book of God: A Response to the Bible* (New Haven: Yale University Press, 1988), p. 130.

M

1. Gilbert K. Chesterton, *Orthodoxy* (London: John Lane, 1909), p. 32.
2. Brian Incigneri, "Did Jesus' family think him mad? Mark 3:20–35," http://www.ccr.org.au/scripture008.html
3. For a contemporary autobiographical version of this scenario—that is, megalomania manifested by withdrawal from ordinary life, interpreted as madness—see Leonard Roy Frank, "Psychiatry's unholy trinity—fraud, fear and force: A personal account," *Ideas On Liberty*, 52: 23-27 (November), 2002.
4. Bertrand Russell, *Power: A New Social Analysis* (London: George Allen & Unwin, 1938), pp. 9, 270.

5. Ray Monk, *Bertrand Russell: The Ghosts of Madness, 1921-1970* (New York: Free Press, 2001).
6. Anne Frank was liquidated by Nazis. Rosemary Kennedy was lobotomized by psychiatrists.
7. William Bennett, quoted in, R. L. Berke, "Drug chief urges youth: Just say who," *New York Times,* May 19, 1989.
8. Eve Kupersanin, "Committing a loved one can be the best medicine," *Catalyst* (The Treatment Advocacy Center), vol. 3, September/October 2001, pp. 10-11.
9. http://jom-emit.cfpm.org/about.html#editors
10. http://jom-emit.cfpm.org/about.html; http://pespmc1.vub.ac.be/MEMLEX.html
11. http://www.connect.net/mattvest/pltclqts.htm
12. Ann Japenga, "Ordeal of postpartum psychosis," *Los Angeles Times,* February 1, 1987, Part Vl, pp. 1 and 4.
13. "Court holds bipolar disorder is physical," *Psychiatric News,* 23:16-17 (March 4), 1988.
14. Joyce Fairbairn, "A Senator's lament: 'Too many Canadians cannot read the Charter of Rights,'" *Whig-Standard* (Kingston, Ontario), September 16, 1987, p. 11.
15. Norm Ovenden, "Southam literacy survey contains unsettling news for newspaper industry," *Whig-Standard* (Kingston, Ontario), September 17, 1987, p. 10. I wish to thank Mark Barnes for providing these two items.
16. "Great Works of Art Pose Health Threats to Tourists," *Post-Standard* (Syracuse), July 26, 1989, p. D1.
17. Lionel Solursh, "Combat addiction: Post-traumatic stress disorder re-explored," *Psychiatric Journal of the University of Ottawa*, 13: 17-20 (March), 1988, p. 20.
18. "Hospital plans to wean teens from Satanism," *Arkansas Democrat,* September 7, 1989, p. 3A.
19. D. C. Dale and D. D. Federman, editors, *Scientific American Medicine* (New York, WebMD Corp., 2001). I thank Tom Rosko, M.D. for calling my attention to this reference.
20. Burkhard Bilger, "Waiting for ghosts: The many careers of Joe Nickell, paranormal investigator," *New Yorker*, December 23 and 30, 2002, pp. 86-100; pp. 88, 95.
21. Jean-Paul Sartre, *No Exit* [1944], in *No Exit and Three Other Plays*, translated by Stuart Gilbert (New York: Knopf, 1948), p. 47.
22. See E.R.L. Gaughran, "From superstition to science: The History of a bacterium," *Transactions of the New York Academy of Sciences,* Series II, 30: 3-24 (Jan.), 1969. For details, see Thomas Szasz, "Introduction," in *Heresies* (New York: Doubleday/Anchor, 1976), pp. 1-22. Also, Ruth Gledhill, "Body of Christ wafers sacrilege," *Times* (London), March 10, 2001, Internet edition; Lauren F. Winner, "Killing Jesus all over again: How medieval stories about desecrating the Eucharist were used to justify the murder of Jews," *Books & Culture*, May/June 2001, http://www.christianitytoday.com/bc/2001/003/10.24.html; "Messages from Heaven," members.aol.com/bjw1106/marian9.htm - 8k; "Daniel Sanford's Miraculous Host Page: Welcome to the Burning & Bleeding Host of Betania," http://dsanford.com/miraclehost.html
23. Richard Weaver, *Ideas Have Consequences* (Chicago: University of Chicago Press /Phoenix Books, 1962).
24. Lewis Wolpert, "Happier off the analyst's couch," *The Sunday Times* (London), February 14, 1999, p. 6/4, emphasis added.
25. Scott Moyers, "Mental patient asks for jury to set him free," *Southeast Missourian*, December 5, 2002, http://www.semissourian.com/story.html$rec=95351; and Fred A. Baughman Jr., "Rodney Yoder—Observations from the trial," December 4, 2002; personal communication from Fred A. Baughman, M.D., board certified neurologist.

26. Thomas Hobbes, *Leviathan* [1651], edited by Michael Oakeshott (New York: Macmillan/Collier, 1962), p. 62.
27. Samuel Butler, *The Way of All Flesh* [1903] (Baltimore: Penguin, 1953), p. 278.
28. Examples abound. See Peter R. Breggin, *Toxic Psychiatry: Why Therapy, Empathy, and Love Must Replace the Drugs, Electroshock, and Biochemical Theories of the "New Psychiatry"* (New York: St. Martin's Press, 1991); Edward Dolnick, *Madness on the Couch: Blaming the Victim in the Heyday of Psychoanalysis* (New York: Simon and Schuster, 1998); Joyce Milton, *The Road to Malpsychia: Humanistic Psychology and Our Discontents* (San Francisco: Encounter Books, 2002); Robert Whitaker, *Mad in America: Bad Science, Bad Medicine, and the Enduring Mistreatment of the Mentally Ill* (New York: Perseus Books, 2001).
29. When a nation represents a fully "monoconfessional Orthodox community, it can in a certain sense be regarded as the one community of faith, an Orthodox nation." Bases of Social Concept of the Russian Orthodox Church, http://216.239.57.100/search?q=cache:EwM3esbLkoAC:www.ortodoks.no/hlolga/ortodoks/doc_no/kirkenidag/social_consept.doc+monoconfessional&hl=en&ie=UTF-8. Although the term "monoconfessional" is used regularly in religious texts, it is listed in neither the *Oxford International Dictionary* nor in *Webster's Third New International Dictionary*.
30. Thomas Szasz, "The myth of mental illness," *American Psychologist*, 15: 113-118 (February), 1960; and *The Myth of Mental Illness: Foundations of a Theory of Personal Conduct* [1961], revised edition (New York: HarperCollins, 1974).
31. *Stacy v. Jones*, "Patents: Chemical for diagnosis of mental ailments," *New York Times*, January 2, 1988, p. B17.
32. William Shakespeare, *A Midsummer Night's Dream*, Act 5, scene 1, lines 15-17.
33. Quoted in Sander L. Gilman, "The Image of the Hysteric," in Sander L. Gilman et al., *Hysteria Beyond Freud* (Berkeley: University of California Press, 1993), pp. 345-452; p. 436.
34. See note 22.

P

1. Sylvia Nasar, *A Beautiful Mind* (New York: Simon and Schuster, 1998). See also Tara Elgin Holley, with Joe Holley, *My Mother's Keeper: A Daughter's Memoir of Growing Up in the Shadow of Schizophrenia* (New York: William Morrow, 1997).
2. "Dismissed alcoholic worker ruled a victim of handicap," *New York Times*, March 4, 1988, p. B9.
3. Thomas S. Szasz, *Ceremonial Chemistry: The Ritual Persecution of Drugs, Addicts, and Pushers* [1974] (Syracuse: Syracuse University Press, 2003), p. 139.
4. C. S. Lewis, *The Business of Heaven: Daily Readings from C. S. Lewis*, edited with a preface by Walter Hooper (New York: Harcourt Brace Jovanovich, 1984), p. 54.
5. Quoted in Tibor Szamuely, *The Russian Tradition*, Robert Conquest, editor (New York: McGraw-Hill, 1974), p. 3.
6. Thomas Jefferson, "Inauguration Address," March 4, 1801, in H. A Washington, editor, *The Writings of Thomas Jefferson* (Philadelphia: Lippincott, 1871), Vol. VIII, Part 11, pp. 1-5; p. 3.
7. Malcolm Lader, *Psychiatry on Trial* (Harmondsworth: Penguin, 1977), pp. 68-69.
8. http://home.earthlink.net/~jehdjh/quotes.html
9. Adam Liptak, "State can make inmate sane enough to execute, court rules," *New York Times*, February 11, 2003. http://www.nytimes.com/2003/02/11/national/11DEAT.html?ex=1045968718&ei=1&en=1b634c5aa71e288c

10. Quoted in Jean Orieux, *Voltaire*, translated by Barbara Bray and Helen R. Lane (Garden City, NY: Doubleday, 1979), p 349.
11. Randolph Bourne, *The Radical Will: Selected Writings, 1911-1918* (New York: Urizen Books, 1977), p. 360.
12. E. Fuller Torrey, quoted in Stephanie Stapleton, "Grey matter?" *American Medical News*, 45: 21-22 (August 19), 2002.
13. Thomas Szasz, "The Lying Truths of Psychiatry," in Ronald Duncan and Miranda Weston-Smith, editors, *Lying Truths: A Critical Scrutiny of Current Beliefs and Conventions* (London: Pergamon Press, 1979), pp. 121-142.
14. Deborah Sontag, "When Politics Is Personal," *New York Times Magazine*, September 15, 2002. http://www.nytimes.com/2002/09/15/magazine/15DOMENIT.html?ex=1032974280&ei=1&en=0f8a45faf7a37fc0
15. Lewis L. Judd, quoted in Ronald Kotulak, "Brain storms: Phenomenal advances in medicine peeling away the secrets of the mind," *Syracuse Herald-journal*, May 23, 1988, pp. B1 and B3; p. B3.
16. Ambrose Bierce, *The Devil's Dictionary* [1911] (New York: Dover, 1958), p. 57.
17. "Surviving spouses' depression studied," *American Medical News,* February 3, 1989, p. 37.
18. Kenneth Minogue, *Alien Powers: The Pure Theory of Ideology* (New York: St. Martin's Press, 1985), p. 5.
19. Sigmund Freud, "Letter to Wilhelm Fliess," February 4, 1888, in Jeffrey Moussaieff Masson, editor, *The Complete Letters of Sigmund Freud to Wilhelm Fliess, 1887-1904* (Cambridge Harvard University Press, 1985), p. 18.
20. Anna Freud, "Letter to Sigmund Freud," July 20, 1922, *Freud Collection*, Library of Congress, quoted in Peter Gay, *Freud: A Life for Our Time* (New York: Norton, 1988), p. 438.
21. Sigmund Freud, "Letter to Wilhelm Fliess," February 1, 1890, in Jeffrey Moussaieff Masson, editor, *The Complete Letters of Sigmund Freud to Wilhelm Fliess, 1887-1904* (Cambridge: Harvard University Press, 1985), p. 398.
22. Sigmund Freud, "Letter to Marie Bonaparte," August 13, 1937, in Ernst L. Freud, editor, *Letters of Sigmund Freud*, translated by Tania and James Stern (New York: Basic Books, 1960), p. 436.
23. Erik Baard, "New science raises the specter of a world without regret: The guilt-free soldier," *Village Voice*, January 22 - 28, 2003. http://www.villagevoice.com/issues/0304/baard.php
24. Quoted in Joan Arehart-Treichel, "Evidence is in: Psychotherapy changes the brain," *Psychiatric News*, 36: 33 (July 6), 2001.
25. Quoted at http://www.toinspire.com/author.asp?author=Goethe. In 1940, Winston Churchill "told a listless nation it was heroic, and it became so." Alistair Cooke, "The Prime Minister was the patient," review of *Churchill At War, 1940-1945*, by Lord Moran, *Wall Street Journal Europe*, December 18, 2002, p. 13.
26. Samuel Butler, *The Way of All Flesh* [1903] (London: Penguin, 1950); Joseph Breuer and Sigmund Freud, *Studies on Hysteria* (1893-95), in *The Standard Edition of the Complete Psychological Works of Sigmund Freud*, edited by James Strachey (London: Hogarth, 1955), Vol. 11.
27. Samuel Butler, *The Way of All Flesh,* pp. 214-215.
28. Sigmund Freud, "Postscript to the Question of Lay Analysis" [1927], in *The Standard Edition of the Complete Psychological Works of Sigmund Freud*, edited by James Strachey (London: Hogarth, 1955), Vol. 20, pp. 255-56.
29. Voltaire, *Philosophical Dictionary*, edited and translated by Theodore Besterman (Harmondsworth: Penguin, 1971), p 289.

30. Hank Briody, "Ask the incarcerated about the death penalty," (Letters), *New York Times*, September 13, 1987, p. E34.
31. Thomas Szasz, "The Socrates option," *Reason*, 24: 47 (April), 1992.

R

1. Alvin Poussaint, quoted in, "Is extreme racism a mental illness?" *The New Crisis*, January-February, 2000, pp. 23-25; p. 23, emphasis added; see also, Alvin Poussaint, "They hate. They kill. Are they insane?" *New York Times*, August 26, 1999. Internet edition.
2. James Earl Jones, quoted in "Jones: American blacks lack unifying language," *The Post-Standard* (Syracuse), October 18, 2000, p. A2.
3. Samuel A. Cartwright, "Report on the diseases and physical peculiarities of the Negro race," *New Orleans Medical and Surgical Journal*, 7: 691-715, 1851; and Thomas Szasz, "The sane slave: An historical note on the use of medical diagnosis as justificatory rhetoric," *American Journal of Psychotherapy*, 25: 228-239 (April), 1971.
4. Stuart Sutherland, *Irrationality: Why We Don't Think Straight* (New Brunswick, NJ: Rutgers University Press, 1992), p. 162.
5. Christopher Longuet-Higgins, "N. S. Sutherland, 1927-1998," November 1998, http://www.biols.susx.ac.uk/EP/stuart.html
6. For example: "Al-Ashari [a tenth-century Islamic scholar] was a literalist…he accepted literally the statements that God has hands and that he sits upon a throne." In Geoffrey Parrinder, editor, *World Religions: From Ancient History to the Present* (New York: Facts on File, 1983), p. 488.
7. "10 die in 4 weeks on Matterhorn," *New York Times*, August 12, 1990.
8. Friedrich A. Hayek, *The Constitution of Liberty* (Chicago: University of Chicago Press, 1960), p. 206.

S

1. Donald C. Goff, "A 23-year-old man with schizophrenia," *JAMA*, 287: 3249-3257 (June 26), 2002, emphasis added.
2. *NAMI E-News,* April 19, 2002, Vol. 02-66. nami-e-news-owner@nami.apollonian.com
3. Editorial, "Why You Can't Buy Insurance," *Wall Street Journal*, October 1, 2002. http://online.wsj.com/article/0, SB1033433111185654113.djm,00
4. Mindy Lewis, *Life Inside: A Memoir* (New York: Atria Books/Simon and Schuster, 2002), p. 334.
5. Editorial, "Embryos and Parkinson's disease," *The Lancet*, 1:1077-1087 (May 14), 1988.
6. Thomas Szasz, *Insanity: The Idea and Its Consequences* [1987] (Syracuse: Syracuse University Press, 1997), p. 365.
7. Joseph Story, *Commentaries on the Constitution of the United States* [1833] (Book 111, chap. XLIV, para. 1877), quoted in George T. Miller, *Religious Liberty in America: History and Prospects* (Philadelphia: Westminster Press, 1976), p. 77.
8. Kenneth L. Woodward, *Making Saints: How the Catholic Church Determines Who Becomes a Saint, Who Doesn't, and Why* (New York: Simon and Schuster, 1990).
9. Myre Sim, "Organic or functional?" *Proceedings of the Royal College of Physicians of Edinburgh*, 17: 232-246 (October), 1987; p. 233.
10. Nigel Hawkes, "Why women have sex on the brain," *Times* (London), September 8, 2001, Internet edition.

11. http://www.standardofcare.com/about/index.html
12. http://www.scarlettlawgroup.com/professional_modern_principles.html
13. "Lawyers back aid in suicide," *New York Times,* September 23, 1987, p. D30.
14. Jay C. Carlisle and Jonathan A. Weiss, "When a client threatens suicide: A lawyer's duty not to disclose," *The New York Professional Responsibility Report*, September 2001, pp. 1-3; p. 3.

T

1. Claudia Dreyfus, "A conversation with Steven Wise: A Courtroom Champion for 4-Legged Creatures," *New York Times*, October 1, 2002. http://www2.verisign-direct.com/pop/dotname/?code=P42C313S1N0B51A8D310V100
2. Thomas S. Szasz, *Law, Liberty, and Psychiatry*: *An Inquiry Into the Social Uses of Mental Health Practices* (New York: Macmillan, 1963), p. 212.
3. Thomas Szasz, "The myth of mental illness," *American Psychologist*, 15: 113-118 (February), 1960; and *The Myth of Mental Illness: Foundations of a Theory of Personal Conduct* [1961], revised edition (New York: HarperCollins, 1974).
4. Thomas Szasz, *Law, Liberty, and Psychiatry: An Inquiry Into the Social Uses of Mental Health Practices* [1963] (Syracuse: Syracuse University Press, 1989), pp. 212-222.
5. Thomas Szasz, *Ceremonial Chemistry: The Ritual Persecution of Drugs, Addicts, and Pushers* [1974] (Syracuse: Syracuse University Press, 2003), p. 139.
6. See *Monomedicine*.
7. Quoted with approval in V. Herzlich and J. Pierret, *Illness and Self in Society* [1984], translated by Elborg Forster (Baltimore: Johns Hopkins, University Press, 1987), p. 231, emphasis added.
8. U.S. Department of Health and Human Services, *The Medicare Handbook* (Baltimore Health Care Financing Administration, Publication No. HCFA 10050, 1980), p. 10.
9. Lord Byron (George Noel Gordon, 1788-1824), *Don Juan: Canto the First*, Stanza CXXXII. http://www.geocities.com/Athens/Acropolis/7389/canto1b.html
10. Samuel Butler (1835-1902), *Erewhon, Or: Over the Range* [1872] (Harmondsworth: Penguin, 1954), pp. 72, 74-75.
11. Samuel Butler, *Erewhon Revisited* [1901], in *Erewhon and Erewhon Revisited* (London: Everyman's Library/J. M. Dent, 1947), p. 242.
12. David Healy, *The Creation of Psychopharmacology* (Cambridge: Harvard University Press, 2002), dust jacket text.
13. H. G. Wells (Herbert George Wells, 1866-1946), *Men Like Gods* (London: Cassell and Company, 1923), pp. 57-58, emphasis added.
14. C. S. Lewis (1898-1963), *The Abolition of Man* [1947] (New York: Macmillan, 1967), pp. 74-77, emphasis in the original.
15. C. S. Lewis, "The humanitarian theory of punishment" [1953], in C. S. Lewis, *God in the Dock: Essays on Theology and Ethics*, edited by Walter Hooper (Grand Rapids, MI: William B. Eerdmans, 1970), pp. 287-294; pp. 292-293.
16. Aldous Huxley (1894-1963), *Brave New World Revisited* [1958] (New York: HarperPerennial, 1989), pp. 81-82.
17. Adolfo Bioy Casares (1914-1999), "Plans for an escape to Carmelo," *New York Review of Books*, April 10, 1986, p. 7.
18. Quoted in *Sexual Medicine Today*, November 1979, p. 19.
19. Timothy E. Quill, Christine K. Cassel, and Diane E. Meier, "The care of the hopelessly ill: Proposed clinical criteria for physician-assisted suicide," *New England Journal of Medicine*, 327: 1380-1384 (November 5), 1992, p. 1381.

V

1. Sheryl Gay Stolberg, "War, murder and suicide: A year's toll is 1.6 million," *New York Times*, October 3, 2002. http://www.nytimes.com/2002/10/03/international/03VIOL.html

Name Index

Subject Index